i

No more STRESS

Your guide to proactive stress management

Written by Davida van der Walt

Edited by Marie Vlok-Sorour
January 2017

Dedicated to my husband and my mother who stood by me through thick and thin when I was diagnosed with Graves Disease.

For information contact:
Davida van der Walt
Davida@ownerteamconsult.com

Foreword

We all have only one life to live and should optimally use the time and opportunities we have available. Most of us, however, fail to achieve continuous growth and the development of our given talents. This is due mainly to an ever-changing environment and the personal demands we are continuously facing.

The present working environment and technology with all its advantages, force us to be available 24/7 and more and more people fall victim to burnout. It is difficult to find balance in our lives and we compromise our health by neglecting to exercise, sleep adequately and eat healthy food – not to even mention making time for ourselves and forging good relationships.

In this timely and important contribution Davida van der Walt provides a practical guide to proactively manage stress and prevent burnout.

Otto Pepler
Life Coach
Johannesburg

January, 2017

Typical Lifestyle Challenges

Falling into a negative thought trap

Have you ever felt so overwhelmed by your circumstances that you were numbed by the experience? Feeling helpless and frustrated! I bet you never paused to examine your thoughts. It is my guess that one negative thought led to the next. And before you knew it, you were in a deep dark pit.

Taking time out is a luxury – autopilot is the norm

Are you running from point A to B, not taking the time to reflect on your priorities? Are you constantly operating on autopilot as it is the only way you can get through each day? Where on earth will you find time for yourself? That's life!

Everyone expects everything from me

Do you constantly feel under pressure? Everyone wants a piece of you. And if you do not deliver, you feel guilty, which compounds the problem. In other words, you add to the pressure.

Stuck in traffic

We are often caught up in traffic, driving anything from one to three hours to get to the office only 30 kilometres away. This can be very stressful. Besides constantly exposing you to exhaust fumes, which are extremely toxic, it taps your energy before you even get to the office.

Technology is taking over our lives

Due to technological advancements and an increasingly globalised work front, we need to be available 24/7. Not to mention social media! We have so many social media mechanisms which we need to keep an eye on, many of which we now also use for work purposes. A few minutes of peace and quiet are an unknown luxury.

When do you want me to exercise?

We all know exercise is important to keep healthy. But where do we find the time? We leave home in the dark, get back home when it is dark... and then work comes home with us. Then there are the challenges at home: making dinner, helping the kids with homework, spending time with the spouse... it is all too much.

Fast food mentality

In the context of our fast-paced lives, we fall into the trap of a fast food mentality. Unfortunately, this means almost everything we consume is processed or chemically enhanced. When we try to be healthy by eating fruit and vegetables, it is covered in pesticides (without our being aware of it). And the meat we eat is pumped full of hormones. Then we try and buy some supposedly healthy snacks which read gluten-free, but when we look at the label, it is full of sugar and chemicals. What is the solution?

We cope by being on a constant adrenaline high

Our bodies are designed to deal with stress by secreting adrenaline. Unfortunately, by design our lives have become such that we never slow down. The body needs recovery time which we are never afforded. When adrenaline does not sustain us, we take energy drinks or one coffee after another. The problem is that at some point the body will retaliate and come to a resounding halt.

Lack of sleep

For the body to recover effectively and the liver to excrete toxins effectively, we need enough sleep, and especially Rapid Eye Movement (REM) sleep. Due to many reasons, we do not sleep enough, or have low quality sleep. One reason is that we sleep with our phones right next to our beds. Cell phones and other electronic equipment, such as tablets and televisions, give off what is known as blue light. Blue light can inhibit the production of the sleep-inducing hormone melatonin and disrupt our sleeping patterns.

We are our own worst enemies

To achieve sustainable health, we need to have a clear vision as to what we want from life and how we will go about it. We tend to float in life's ocean without a clear strategy to achieve our goals, or even without clear goals. Because we lack clarity on our goals and priorities, we convince ourselves that everything is important and we try and please everyone. False guilt kicks in and we stretch ourselves to the limit.

We lose sight of what is important in life. We build our house on sand instead of rock!

In this book, I hope to provide you with practical guidance on how to develop a strategy and plan for your life that is achievable and sustainable, that will guide you to happiness, a sense of achievement and health.

It all starts with knowing what you want from life, what is important, and then taking accountability to make it happen!

Preface

Introduction

The purpose of this book is to provide you with practical advice on how to focus your energy to prevent burnout and achieve sustainable health through proactive stress management. Health in this context implies physical and emotional health.

The foundation of this book was developed in 2007 after I experienced burnout and decided to take on the challenge to develop a life strategy process to help myself and others in the pursuit of sustainable health. Then in 2015 I was diagnosed with an autoimmune disease, which at the time felt like a death sentence. I went back to my life strategy material and dusted it off. Using those same principles and doing further research on how to naturally strengthen the immune system, I now feel confident to share the fundamentals of sustainable health with you. My passion is to make people aware of how toxic their lives are and what they can do about it. My vision is to share what I have learned with as many people as possible and ultimately to make a significant impact on the quality of life of people across the globe.

This book will guide you to proactively manage the impact of stress on your life.

For whom is the book intended?

This book is aimed at any one who is either seeing the signs of burnout or is already experiencing the disastrous effects of burnout. But it is also for those who feel that their lives are not going anywhere. If you feel like a boat floating aimlessly in the middle of the ocean, then this book is for you.

Layout of the book

The book comprises 9 chapters.

Chapter 1 contextualises stress.

Chapter 2 describes the various stressors we are exposed to and challenges you to take a good look at your life and to raise your awareness of your specific stressors.

Chapter 3 considers the symptoms of stress and allows you to reflect on how stress is affecting you.

Chapter 4 provides an overview of the four keys to avoiding burnout and achieving sustainable health.

Chapters 4, 5, 6 and 7 unpack the various keys to avoiding burnout, namely detoxing your mind, detoxing your environment, detoxing your body and building your house on a Rock.

Chapter 8 considers how you can make change last by developing solid habits.

Chapter 9 provides guidance on how to make these significant life changes last.

About the author

Davida van der Walt

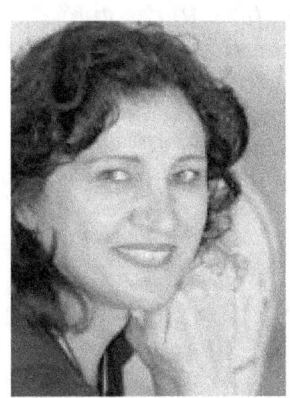

I am an industrial psychologist with a passion for wellness. Besides my experience addressing the softer issues on projects, I facilitate life strategy workshops and conduct life coaching where I share the principles captured in this book.

My personal experience with an autoimmune disease and recovering from it to the extent that I am in remission, puts me in a unique position to share what works and what doesn't.

My aim is to empower you to take charge of your life, your thoughts, your decisions and your health. I read many health journals and sometimes must read an article five times to know exactly what it is about. My aim is to write this book in simple terms and language that everyone can understand, regardless of their background. I sincerely hope that you find this book of interest and that it provides you with the tools to take responsibility for your life and health.

Davida van der Walt

May 2017

What experts say

"This book is a "must-read" for all of us stressed South Africans. Davida van der Walt has done an outstanding job at simplifying a medically complex ailment. Her practical questionnaires make it easy for us to self-diagnose whether we are suffering from Stress and Burnout. Her practical step by step guidance on how to resolve these stresses allows for easy and sustainable interventions for detoxifying your emotions, body and environment. Most of all I really value her guidance of how to identify our purpose and change our behavior so that we are able to manage our stressors effectively. I highly recommend this book as it is likely to change your ability to cope with stress forever."

Dr. Dhesan G. Moodley
MMed Sc Metabolic Nutritional Medicine (USF), MMed Sport Science (UCT), MbChB (UKZN), MBA (UCT)

Table of Contents

Chapter 1- Burnout in Context

"Burnout is what happens when you try to avoid being human for too long." Michael Gungor

Introduction

Do you need this book?

Let us start off with a quick self-assessment:
1. Do you take a painkiller or muscle relaxant almost every day to deal with your aches and pains?
2. Do you wake up tired and go to bed tired?
3. Do you feel tense or anxious most of the time?
4. Do you fall ill easily?
5. Are you busy all the time, yet feel as if you are not achieving much?
6. Do you always have an excuse not to exercise?
7. Are you so busy that you do not have time to cook healthy meals?
8. Are your relationships suffering because you can't get to everything that is important?
9. Does your life feel meaningless?

Watch out! You might be headed for burnout and once you've let yourself go that far, you may never be the same again. If you are already at burnout, make sure to read this book carefully. There is hope!

If you answered yes to any one of these questions, you need to read this book. If you answered yes to four or more of these questions, I suggest you don't let go until you finished reading every chapter and completed all the exercises. Do not think that by only reading it you have done your part. Take the time and complete the exercises. You won't regret it.

To start off, let's understand burnout and its consequences.

Burnout in context

What is burnout? Burnout is a type of psychological stress. It is characterised by exhaustion, lack of enthusiasm, lack of motivation, feelings of ineffectiveness, frustration and cynicism. It results in reduced efficacy at home and in the workplace.

Burnout is thus a state of emotional, physical, social, and spiritual exhaustion. It can lead to compromised health, social withdrawal, depression and a spiritual malaise. Often burnout is the result of an extended period of exertion at a particular task (generally with no obvious payoff or end in sight) or of carrying too many burdens. It can also be the result of self-reliance – trying to retain control over everyone and everything. It is the result of overwhelming demands or responsibilities, either placed on us by others or by ourselves.

The risk of burnout is that it can cause long-term chemical changes in your body that remain even after you feel better. These changes make you more vulnerable to stress and to contracting diseases like colds and flu. People who have suffered physical symptoms from stress should continue whatever stress management interventions they used to help themselves recover, even after they feel better.

The burnout curve is depicted in Figure 1.

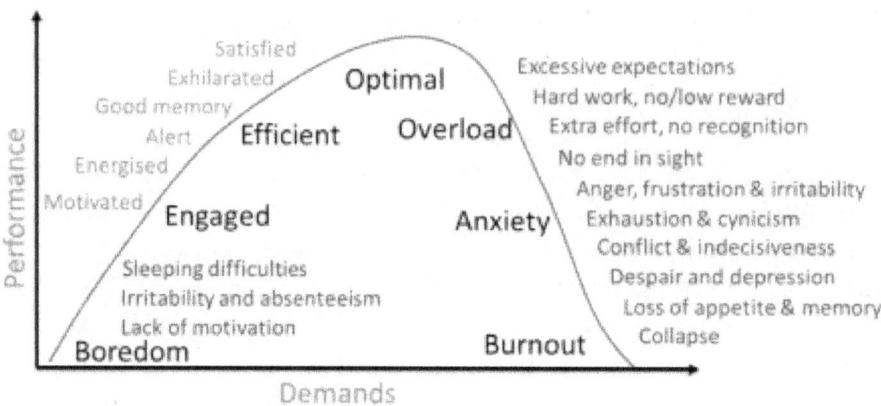

Figure 1: The Burnout Curve

To understand burnout, stress must be seen in context. Stress is a state of mental or emotional strain or tension resulting from adverse or demanding circumstances. It must be seen in relation to the demands you are faced with as depicted in Figure 1. It then directly impacts your performance and if the demands are too many or too intense for too long, it can lead to burnout.

All types of stress are not by default bad! Stress can also enhance performance. Positive stress is referred to as eustress, while negative stress is referred to as distress. It is very interesting that if the demands in your life and in the workplace, are too low, it also causes distress.

As can be seen in the Burnout Curve, if you are underutilised and not exposed to demands in line with your abilities, you will be bored, which will lead to sleeping difficulties, irritability, absenteeism and lack of motivation. But if you are exposed to demands aligned with your abilities and capacity, you will be engaged, efficient and function optimally at the top of the curve. Then you will feel motivated, energised and alert, display good memory and feel exhilarated and satisfied. Once the demands exceed that optimal level, and the pressure becomes too much, overload and anxiety sets in, which ultimately leads to burnout. In this process, you are exposed to excessive expectations and demands, either from others or yourself. You will put in a lot of effort, but will not feel that you are getting the reward for your hard work. Then you will try even harder and work even longer hours, which will exacerbate the feeling that you are not recognised for what you do. It will start to feel that there is no end in sight, which will culminate in major frustration, irritability and anger. You will start to feel exhausted and cynical. As the pressure mounts, you will become indecisive and experience conflict in relationships. Despair, depression and loss of appetite will set in. In some cases, it culminates in an increased appetite. You will start to forget even the smallest little detail. You will walk into a room to get something and will get there not knowing what you were looking for. And before you know it, you will collapse. Collapse is the final stage of burnout.

Shirra Moch is a lecturer in the Department of Pharmacy, Pharmacology and Health Sciences at the University of the Witwatersrand in Johannesburg, South Africa. The focus of her research is stress (Palkhivala, 2015). Moch and her colleagues conducted a study on 16 people who suffered a stress burnout so severe that they had to be hospitalised. She reported that they mostly spent the day in bed, crying. Normally, when peoples' bodies are stressed by an illness, or their minds are stressed by external circumstances or even an argument with a spouse, the body secretes the hormone cortisol. This hormone helps the body fight off disease. Many overstressed people have too much cortisol, but the people Moch studied had low cortisol levels.

Moch's patients were given intensive stress management therapy while they were in hospital, which included medication and courses in meditation, breathing, exercise and nutrition. They also saw a social worker who taught them to handle stressful situations and a psychiatrist who gave them talk therapy. They participated in this programme all day for about five days while in hospital and then half days for a short time after they were discharged. Afterwards, they came in for monthly follow-up sessions.

The intense stress management worked only up to a point. The people with burnout did start to feel better and were able to go back to work and live normal lives. However, their cortisol levels remained low, even after five months. This means they remained more susceptible to diseases like colds and flu and were more likely to have another burnout episode if they didn't adhere to the stress management changes they were taught.

Moch presented these findings at the 32nd Annual Meeting of the International Society of Psychoneuroendocrinology. Moch stated: "When they feel well, they start to backslide right away (on the stress management programme), it's only when they start to feel sick again that they think, 'oh yes, I have to do all this stuff again!' We're trying to educate them that this is lifestyle change."

Making a lifestyle change

Eureka!!! Did you get that! It is a lifestyle change. Lifestyle changes can only come with a commitment to take action!

According to the Concise Oxford Dictionary, commitment is:
- A decision – morally dedicated to a cause;
- Action – doer of;
- Perseverance – pledge oneself by implication to a course of action.

In other words, commitment = decision + action + perseverance.

If you are reading this book with the hope of getting a quick fix and a recipe that will change your life instantly, don't bother. This book is about taking accountability for your life. If you are willing to do so, this book will change your life dramatically for the better.

You will be provided with many tips and tricks that can easily be implemented in your life and that will have an impact on your health and ability to ward off burnout. The only way to beat burnout and to remain happy and healthy is following a holistic approach.

Work-life balance – fact or fiction?

What do you think about work-life balance? Is it achievable?

There are many interesting books on life coaching that try to give us the perfect recipe for finding work-life balance. We need to plan our time well and consequently find time for all the important things in our lives. But we also need to do all those urgent things, burning our backsides ever so gently.

Let me illustrate by giving an example typical of most households. The husband needs to work to provide for his family. But in this day and age, very few wives have the luxury to be stay-at-home moms; consequently, she also works full-time. They juggle to get the kids to school and to attend after-school activities. On top of that they need to make sure the bills are paid, shopping is done, they need to eat healthy food, exercise, spend time with friends and family, remember to buy birthday presents, make sure the house is kept clean, support the children with their homework, etc, etc. Just when they think they have some sort of routine, the car breaks down, or the home computer has a virus, a pipe bursts or grandma falls ill. Never a dull moment!

How do you find balance among all of those? Have you ever heard such nonsense!? Balance! I think if you find a person who has perfect work-life balance, who can juggle all the balls equally well, he or she is more than likely by now checked into some clinic for burnout.

Reality is that all of us have a lot of balls to juggle. This causes stress. What causes even more stress is living for the sake of living. Many of us are just little boats floating in a huge sea. We have no destination. We go where the current takes us. This leads to feelings of worthlessness. We feel hopeless and directionless. Yet lifestyle changes can only be implemented successfully if we know what we want from life and where we want to go. Do you know what your personal vision, your values and passions are? Are you aligning your lifestyle to your vision? I like using the analogy of a band. If they all play to the same tune, beautiful music arises. Or lives are the same. If you know what you want out of life, the different aspects of your life need to play to the same tune. In reality, different aspects of our lives may take priority at different stages of our lives. For example, if you have fallen ill, your work priorities will have to take a back seat. But the one ball you can never drop is your health.

This book will put you on a journey of self-discovery which will help you identify your biggest stressors, realise what they are doing to you, help you identify the stress management techniques that will work for you, and guide you in making lifestyle changes that will be sustainable. We have all made some drastic changes in our lives that we battle to maintain. This resource will give you the skills to make sure that you maintain the changes you implement in your life!

Enough said. Without any further deliberation, let's start the journey...

Chapter 2 - Defining your Stressors

"Burnout is when long exhaustion meets diminished interest." Unknown

Understanding your stressors

We will start by exploring the stressors in every facet of your life. We will also explore how these affect you, and what you can do about them.

Our stressors can be classified into a few main categories namely: career, environmental, psycho-emotional, physiological, relationships, important events that you experienced in the past and your personality type (Chapter 2). When these stressors have a negative impact on you, they could manifest themselves in physical, psycho-emotional and social symptoms (Chapter 3). In Chapter 3 you will complete a few very simple exercises that will help you define your stressors. You will be challenged to take a good look at yourself and to face your stressors head on. Chapter 4 will contextualise the four keys to managing stress proactively and avoiding burnout. Chapters 5-9 will guide you through these keys and how to apply them practically in your life.

What are your stressors?

We are all faced with multiple stressors every day of our lives. You might think that stressors are those things we are exposed to that could potentially have a negative impact on us. Not necessarily. People respond in different ways to stressors. Some are motivated by them, while others may experience extreme symptoms as a result. Stressors are typically divided into five categories: Career/intellectual, environmental, psycho-emotional, physiological and relationship stressors.

Career/Intellectual stressors

Career or intellectual stressors refer to any work or study related stressors. In a negative context, it typically refers to stress that you are being exposed to because your career is not progressing as you anticipated, or your work environment is unsatisfactory.

We all know that in the workplace the only constant is change. Change brings about great stress. You end up not knowing where you are going with your career, when you will get promoted, what you will be doing, and so forth.

In South Africa, an added dynamic is Employment Equity. Some organisations fast track young black professionals. In some instances, some of these young professionals tend to be set up for failure. By moving too fast, their experience levels fall short, rendering them unable to deal with the delicate dynamics in the work environment. They are put under great pressure, which sometimes can have disastrous consequences for both the organisation and the person involved. What saddens me is that in many instances individuals are broken in the process. On the other side of the coin, white South Africans' careers tend to be stifled and job opportunities limited. The spirit of employment equity legislation is sound and well understood, but unfortunately often poorly implemented to the detriment of many, regardless their race.

Given the political scene in South Africa, many people opt for starting their own businesses. In the current climate, you need to be tough to cope with managing your own business. Small business owners will know exactly what I am talking about. Labour legislation and taxation requirements make it almost impossible to run a profitable business. Besides having to deal with labour issues, legislation increasingly brings about greater financial strain on small business owners. Government is introducing legislation to protect employees, but the consequences for the small business owner are not always taken into consideration. From my perspective, small business owners are the one group of people in South Africa which are exposed to the greatest levels of stress.

As you will note later in this book, our aim is to proactively manage our stress to either limit our stressors, or to make sure we are able and strong enough to cope with them. Stress cannot always be avoided, but it can be managed!

Another interesting career stressor is being overloaded or under loaded at work. I guess everyone agrees that if you are overloaded for an extended period, this will eventually lead to burn out. You will become irritable, forgetful and indecisive, which will in turn lead to sleepless nights and strained relationships. On the other hand, if you are underutilised at work, not challenged enough, you will lack motivation, be irritable, have sleeping difficulties and avoid work. The exciting part is that we all have a threshold in terms of our career stress where we can experience optimal stress. Yes! Optimal stress!

When you are exposed to the correct level of stress, you will feel motivated, energised, in control, alert and sometimes exhilarated. I know you know what I am talking about.

Environmental stressors

Environmental stressors refer to any exposure in your work and living environment which is potentially not conducive to your physical or emotional health. The most prevalent stressors in our day and age are overcrowding, traffic, pollution, crime, economic strain, increased electricity rates and power cuts. I guess if a foreigner reads this book, they will have a good laugh. I find it astonishing how much stress the power cuts in South Africa bring about. As we all know, load shedding is a constant threat. This means that everyone gets a chance to be without electricity, in other words, we share the load. Recently water restrictions have also been introduced in some areas.

The effects of power cuts are immeasurable. On an individual level we are inconvenienced. While cooking dinner, and doing the laundry, the power goes off. Some appliances, such as decoders, can be damaged by power cuts. The other consequence is getting stuck in traffic because all the traffic lights are out. You do not want to be in Johannesburg traffic during power cuts. You are sure to be late for your appointment. From a business perspective, it has disastrous implications. Businesses like restaurants can't operate without electricity. It has a significant impact on business profits and ultimately the country's economy.

Crime is another South African reality. As I am in my mid-forties I have been exposed to five house break-ins. I have been mugged and my husband has survived an attempted hi-jacking at gunpoint. Unthinkable! Of all the stressors discussed in this book, the impact of crime is the most severe. Being scared and ready for "action" every moment of every day is stressful. The fight-or-flight response (also called hyper arousal or the acute stress response) is a physiological reaction that occurs in response to a perceived threat. It enables us to survive. Whenever we perceive a physical or psychological threat, an inbuilt reflex or alarm system in our brains triggers the release of electrical impulses and a variety of hormones. There is a complex hormonal cascade of over 30 stress hormones, such as adrenalin, noradrenalin and cortisol, which have a powerful and widespread effect on our bodies' biochemistry, physiology and psychology, giving us the extra strength and speed we need to deal with the threatening situation. The fight-or-flight response was designed for short-term use. Sadly, many of us cope on an extended basis using the fight-or-flight response, which wreaks havoc with our hormones, because our biggest stressors are psycho-emotional. These last for weeks or months or even years on end.

Psycho-emotional stressors

Psycho-emotional stressors refer to any event or activity in our lives that is rooted in our psyche and brings about emotional discomfort. These differ from one person to the next. What creates an emotional response in one person might have no effect on the next.

Psycho-emotional stressors are mainly the result of how people think and feel about themselves, like trying to live up to some expectation and not being able to do so. You may want to look differently, have a different car, job, salary or spouse. It's all about not feeling in control of your life and not accepting yourself for who you are.

Many of us have deep rooted uncertainties and fears which haunt us for life.

Physiological Stressors

Physiological stressors refer to your general health and fitness. When your body is suffering because you are not nourishing it with healthy food, exercising it to stay fit, nor sleeping enough to allow it to recover, you will be stressed. It also includes exposing your body to harmful substances.

Relationship stressors

Relationship stressors are those stressors that relate to all the relationships we have, such as family, friends, co-workers or even ourselves. Are those relationships healthy? Or are they stress inducing?

Analyse your Stressors

The best place to start is to try and understand where you find yourself today in terms of the stressors you expose yourself to. Do note my wording, stressors you expose yourself to. We need to be far more aware of what we put ourselves through. By taking charge, we can greatly reduce our stressors. In the last chapter of this book, I will tell you my story and will share with you how I reduced my stressors, which by the way, is a continuous process.

Stressor Survey

The stressors questionnaire covers most of the stressors we are exposed to in the South African context, but it is also universally applicable. *This questionnaire's sole purpose is to establish the degree or extent to which you are exposed to these stressors.* It does not necessarily consider how these stressors are affecting you. The impacts will follow later. The scoring instructions follow directly after the questionnaire. Five categories of stressors are used, namely career, environmental, psycho-emotional, physiological and relationship stressors.

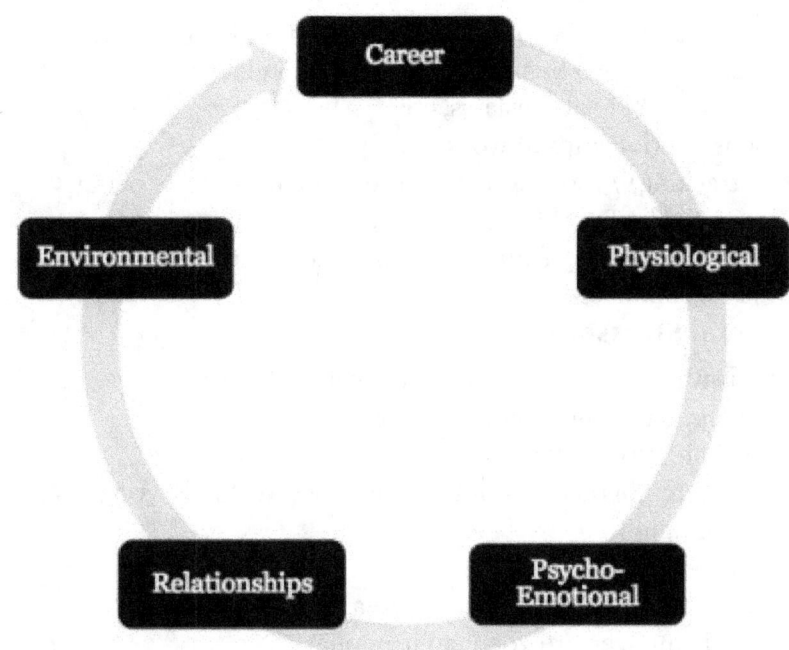

Figure 2: Stressors

Indicate with a tick which of these stressors you are regularly exposed to.

Career Stressors	
Rapid and constant changes at work, e.g. re-organisation, retrenchments, etc	
I manage people that need constant supervision	
Work demands affecting my personal life, e.g. taking work home, working shifts, working long hours, etc	
I am studying part-time while working	
Unsatisfactory remuneration and benefits, financial difficulties	
Underutilisation (bored, no challenges)	
Overloaded at work	

Career Stressors	
I am an entrepreneur with my own business and need to cope with stress of managing my own business and growing legislative requirements (tax, VAT), labour laws, etc	
Conflict or poor relationships at work	
Too fast (fast tracking) / too slow career progression (such as being negatively impacted by Employment Equity)	
Lack of direction/leadership from my management, e.g. role clarification/role confusion	
Environmental Stressors	
Travelling in heavy traffic, being exposed to exhaust fumes	
Crime (hi-jacking, muggings, robberies, etc)	
Air pollution where I work/stay	
Extreme weather/temperature conditions where I work/live (very hot, cold, dry, humid, rainy)	
Noise at work/home	
Water shortage/water restrictions in my area	
Working/living in an over-crowded environment	
Poor working/living conditions	
Power cuts at work/home	
Long distance travelling to work/home (car/taxi/bus/air)	

Psycho-Emotional Stressors	
I feel emotionally abused	
Nobody cares about me	
I lack emotional support due to e.g. poor relations, being far away from my family, etc	
I cannot do much about changing my circumstances	
I am overwhelmed by everything I need to deal with	
I am labelled because of my race/I am single/divorced/gay/overweight, or any other	
I don't like most people	
I don't have anyone that understands me or what I am going through	
I am not happy with me	

Physiological Stressors	
I am unfit	
I use/abuse drugs	
I follow an unbalanced diet (consume a lot of junk/processed food)	
I indulge in "comfort food"	
I don't sleep well	
I am physically abused	
I smoke	
I take medication to relax (e.g. sleeping tablets and/or painkillers)	
I take painkillers on a regular basis	
I neglect my body	
I regularly consume alcohol	
Relationships	
I do not like myself	
I experience inner conflict	
I have strained relations with my partner	
I have strained relationships with my parent/s	
I have strained relationships with my in-laws	
I have strained relationships with my children	
I have strained relationships with my stepchildren/family	
I have strained relationships with my co-workers	
I have a strained relationship with my boss	

Consider all the stressors you marked and decide which of these have a significant negative impact on your life and stress levels. Prioritise them and write the top five in the spaces below.

1. _____
2. _____
3. _____
4. _____
5. _____

No two people are alike and no two people are affected by stress in the same way.

For some stress is a motivator. As said earlier, everyone has an optimal stress level. But once stress levels become excessive, resulting in illness or dysfunctional behaviour, you need to manage it reactively, while putting proactive measures in place to manage, or rather prevent, its effects going into the future.

Take a few minutes to think about the stressors you listed above. Over which of these do you have some level of control? What can **you** change?

The next section considers life events you experienced that impacted your stress levels.

Life events

In the course of your life, there are always events that you either plan for or not, but that inevitably create enormous amounts of stress.

Much research has been done on the relationship between major life events and the onset of illness. The impact of such events is considered cumulative. The more events you experience, the greater the impact and possibility of illness (Rabkin & Elmer, 1976). In their research they found a relationship between mounting life changes and the occurrence of sudden cardiac death, accidents, diabetes, etc. They also found that some people were severely affected by life events and others not. There are multiple factors impacting your ability to cope with life events, some of which include your personality and your ability to maintain a healthy immune system. They indicate that most research done on this topic was based on the original work done by Holmes and Rahe who developed a 43-item checklist. The list below is also an adapted version of the work done by Holmes and Rahe.

You can already get a sense of how important it is to be aware of the life events impacting on you and ensuring that your body is strong enough to fend off life's attacks.

Death of a spouse or a close family member is one of the events that have the greatest impact on any individual. Break up, divorce or marital separation also has a significant impact on a person's stress levels. In my opinion, any direct exposure to crime is as stressful, if not worse, depending on the physical and emotional scars left by the criminal incident. Another major cause of stress is immigration (either you yourself or someone close to you). Immigration is a common phenomenon these days. It does, however, not go without great discomfort.

Below is a list of typical life events. Seeing these in context over time may help you realise how much you have been able to withstand. All of these events are self-explanatory, with the exception of the last one. How can a holiday be stressful? We go on holiday to get rid of all our stress and worries. Let me draw a picture. You and your husband decide to go to his parents at the Coast over Christmas and to your parents for New Year. Your mother is angry at you for not spending Christmas at "home", your in-laws are upset because last year you spent both Christmas and New Year at your folks. On your way to the Coast, you pass an accident scene and get stuck in traffic for more than two hours. As you reach the coast, just before dark, you have a flat tyre. The next day you go to the shops, just to realise that the groceries down at the Coast are double the price than back at home. Then to top it all, after one day of sunshine, it starts raining. It only stops the day before you return home. In the middle of your holiday, you get a call to inform you that a pipe had burst at your house. Sounds familiar? That is what I call stressful!

Are you ready to consider your life events? Go for it! Consider the list below and indicate which of these life events happened to you in the last 6 – 18 months. Indicate which of these have had a major or severe impact on your life and your stress levels? If the event occurred more than 18 months ago, but is still affecting you today, indicate the impact as you experience it today.

Life Events	Major impact	Severe impact
Death of spouse or close family member/friend		
Break-up/divorce/marital separation		
Being directly exposed to crime (e.g. high jacking, break-in, etc)		
Immigrating and adapting to another country / close family member immigrated		
Personal injury/illness or change in health of close family member/friend/miscarriage		
Physical/emotional abuse		
Marriage/getting engaged/marital reconciliation		
Transferred/promoted/retrenched/fired/retired/demoted		
Pregnancy		
Sexual difficulties		
New baby in the family/new family member, e.g. adoption / becoming aware of a relative not previously known		
Change in financial status (up or down)		
Son/daughter/close relative leaving home		
Conflict with parents or in-laws		
Spouse begins/stops work		
Begin or end studies (university/educational institution)		
Change in living conditions (e.g. someone moved in/out)		
Change in personal habits (e.g. stopped smoking)		
Conflict with manager/colleague/subordinate		
Change in work hours/conditions/location		
Change in residence/moving house		
Bought a new house/car		
Vacation/holidays		

Take a few moments to reflect on these life events and indicate below which of these have had the most significant impact on your life from a stress point of view.

1. _____
2. _____
3. _____
4. _____
5. _____

By now you can start seeing the compounding effect of the different stressors in your life, and how your various life events have added to the stress you have been exposed to.

The next section will help you determine whether your personality is a stressor in your life or whether it helps you manage your stress.

Personality

I can just imagine what you are thinking right now. "How can my personality be a stressor?" I have news for you. No matter where you live in the world, personality traits can be our worst enemy as far as stressors are concerned.

The Type A and Type B personality theory had its inception in the 1950s. It describes a pattern of behaviours that was a risk factor for coronary heart disease. This theory has been widely popularised and widely criticised for its scientific shortcomings. But once you have completed this exercise, you will agree that your personality does have an impact on your stress levels. The Type A and B Personality theory places personalities on a continuum. We all know personalities are far more complex than that. But for the sake of understanding yourself, and the extent to which you place pressure on yourself and others, this exercise will suffice.

If you look at the continuum below, where will you plot yourself? Will you be to the far left, in the middle or to the far right?

Type A	Type B
• Never late	• Not concerned with time
• Very competitive	• Not competitive
• Anticipates what others are going to say and interrupts	• Good listener
• Always feels under pressure	• Never feels under pressure
• Impatient	• Patient
• Tries to do many things at once, thinks about what to do next. Perceived as impulsive.	• Tackles life one step at a time
• Fast & forceful	• Takes time talking and formulating ideas
• Pushes self very hard	• Takes time doing things
• Always in a hurry	• Do not push self very hard
• Pushes others to perform	• Never rushed, takes your time
	• Do not push others to perform

Figure 3: Type A and B Personalities and Stress

We are all somewhere on this continuum. Some of us are extreme Type A's and others are extreme Type B's. Some of us lie in the middle, which means we can move to either side as we choose. The higher your level of self-awareness, the better you can manage your personality.

If you are an extreme Type A personality, you would tend to have a sense of time urgency ("Hurry Sickness"), you will be very competitive, impatient, fast and forceful in everything you say and do. You will often feel under pressure. You will experience hostility or anger toward others not performing to your standards.

If you are an extreme Type B personality, you will take your time to do things. You will be patient, take time to talk, express your feelings and never or rarely feel under pressure. You will stay calm and collected under most circumstances.

The main message here is that if you are a Type A personality, you will place a lot of pressure on yourself and others. Your personality thus acts as a stressor in your life. On the other hand, if you are a Type B, you are a relaxed person who is not prone to stress. You will, however, increase the stress levels of a type A person, because you are not moving fast enough. Later in this book we will explore how you can increase your self-awareness and implement tools and techniques to help you manage your personality effectively.

What can we conclude?

Up to this point we looked at possible stressors. We assessed your career, environmental, emotional, physical and relationship stressors, as well as the life events you have been exposed to that may add to your stress. This was followed by your quick and dirty personality assessment.

At this point you should have a clear idea of what your key stressors are.

Before moving on, it is important to once again emphasise that because stress is such a personal experience, the stressors listed may not cover all the stressors relevant to your life. You may have something specific, like having different spiritual beliefs from your spouse, which may be a major stressor. This is but one example of other stressors that could have a severe impact on your life. An attempt was made to cover the typical stressors experienced by most people.

Take a few moments to consider whether there are any other significant stressors in your life which have not been covered up to this point.

To conclude this chapter, make a short list of your main stressors that you need to address.

1. _____
2. _____
3. _____
4. _____
5. _____

In the next chapter we will consider the impact of stress on your life. By understanding both your stressors and how they impact you, you will find yourself in a position to take charge and do something about it.

Chapter 3 - Symptoms of Stress

"In dealing with those who are undergoing great suffering, if you feel "burnout" setting in, if you feel demoralised and exhausted, it is best for the sake of everyone, to withdraw and restore yourself. The point is to have a long-term perspective." Dalai Lama

What are the symptoms of stress?

Some people cope well with stress, others don't. We are all unique in terms of how we respond to the stressors we covered in Chapter 2. What we do have in common is that stress becomes visible through one or more symptom(s). We often mistake these stress symptoms for some form of illness. Even though it may be classified as an illness, it is caused by stress.

The exciting news is that if you are able to identify which of your symptoms are stress related and pinpoint the source of the stress, you can actually do something about it.

The whole aim of this book is to create a level of self-awareness which will put you in a position of power. You will know what is happening to you, why it is happening and what you can do about it. In essence we are talking about proactive stress management.

Up to now we have looked at the possible sources of stress. Now we will consider the symptoms of stress. Generally the negative symptoms of stress can be categorised in groups, namely: physical, psycho-emotional and social.

Physical

When we experience stress, our bodies respond with a fight-or-flight response as mentioned in Chapter 1. This has a negative impact on our immune systems. It manifests itself in physical symptoms such as headaches, migraine, backache, allergies, fatigue, exhaustion, indigestion, sexual dysfunction, high blood pressure and so forth.

Psycho-emotional

Over and above the physical symptoms, psycho-emotional symptoms come into play. We have all experienced these and possibly do right now. Psycho-emotional symptoms include impatience, frustration, sleeping difficulties, loss of emotional control and lack of concentration. Psychological and emotional responses to stress are typically intertwined.

Social

The frustration of dealing with the physical and the psycho-emotional symptoms has a social impact. Some social symptoms include being over worked, becoming quiet, reckless driving, eating more or less than usual, expression of anger, impatience with others, taking time off work and road rage, to mention a few.

These symptoms are often coinciding. Some people experience greater physical symptoms because they may suppress their emotions. In most cases, however, the symptoms in one area tend to spill over into the other. The next questionnaire brings us to the point of facing the extent to which the stressors identified so far actually affect you. Let's look at which symptoms you experience as a result of the stress you are exposed to. Complete the survey below.

Indicate which of these symptoms you experience regularly or all the time:

Physical Symptoms of Stress	
Fatigue/exhaustion/tiredness	
Heart palpitations	
Allergies/acute sinus/asthma	
Painful jaw/headache as result of grinding teeth	
Muscle spasms, e.g. neck ache/back ache	
Headache/migraine	
Hot flushes/cold sweats	
Sweaty hands and feet	
Stomach irregularities/indigestion	
Dizziness/unsteadiness	
Psycho-emotional Symptoms of Stress	
Impatience	
Difficulty concentrating	
Difficulty relaxing	
Mood swings	
Anxiety	
Frustration/easily angered	
Feelings of detachment	
Racing thoughts	
Sleeping difficulties	
Emotional outbursts	
Social Symptoms of Stress	
Drown yourself in a specific activity, e.g. work, games, etc	
Become quiet	
Easily irritated or annoyed with others	
Sexual difficulties	
Aggression	
Eat more/less than usual	
Smoke/drink more than usual	
Drive recklessly	
Impatient with family and friends	
Self-isolation, withdraws from social interaction	

These symptoms cannot be ignored. What did you you learn from your answers? Which category dominates? Physical, psycho-emotional or social? Does the one impact the other?

Which of these concerns you most? Now is the time to be honest with yourself.

Capture the five most concerning symptoms below:

1. _____
2. _____
3. _____
4. _____
5. _____

What can we conclude?

By now you will have a clear picture of where you are in terms of your various stressors, but more importantly, how they affect you. You can also now draw parallels between the symptoms you experience. If you are constantly fatigued, your immune system is taking strain, which means more than likely you are suffering with aches, pains and allergies. These in turn affect your sleep patterns, which will impact your anxiety levels. Due to your high frustration levels, you are likely to be annoyed with others and to cope, you may eat or drink more than usual to calm you down.

This is a vicious circle! The good news is you can do something about it!

Half the battle is won by having an acute awareness of what your stressors are and how they affect you. This information will empower you to make the changes you need to be happy and healthy!

The question that now remains is: "Do you want to do something about it?" If the answer is yes, please do not stop reading. This book will change your life.

Chapter 4 - The four keys to avoiding burnout and achieving sustainable health

"The best six doctors anywhere, and no one can deny it, are sunshine, water, rest, air, exercise and diet."
Wayne Fields

A holistic and proactive approach

There is no one recipe that will work for everyone in dealing with their stressors. We are all unique creatures with a unique make-up. What may severely impact one of us, may have no impact on someone else. Therefore, it was very important that you took the time to carefully read through Chapters 1 to 3 and completed all exercises.

Following a holistic approach in dealing with your stress is the only long-term and sustainable solution.

The specifics of what may work for you will be different from the person next to you, yet some principles are universal. Figure 1 contains the four keys to avoiding burnout and ensuring sustainable health. In this chapter, we will briefly look at each of these keys namely detoxing the mind, detoxing the body, detoxing the environment and building your house on a Rock. In the following chapters, we will unpack these keys in greater detail.

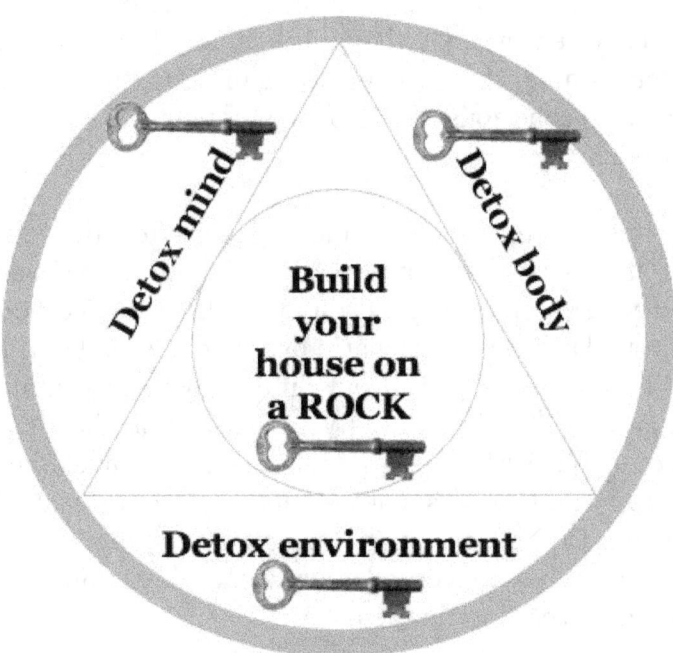

Figure 3: Proactive Stress Management

Detox your mind

Let's start with detoxing the mind. What does that mean? It means you must rid your mind of all negative, toxic thoughts.

Dr Caroline Leaf states on her website that "75% to 95% of the illnesses that plague us today are a direct result of our thought life. What we think about affects us physically and emotionally. It's an epidemic of toxic emotions." She states that the average person has over 30,000 thoughts a day. If these thoughts go unchecked, a breeding ground for illness is created. In other words, we make ourselves sick. Dr Leaf on her website quotes research that shows that fear, all on its own, triggers more than 1,400 known physical and chemical responses and activates more than 30 different hormones. Toxic waste (generated by toxic thoughts) causes illnesses such as diabetes, cancer, asthma, skin problems and allergies, to name just a few. She urges us to consciously control our thought life and to start detoxing our brains.

Let's explore this concept for a moment. How often do you ask yourself what if this or that happened, what could have been if circumstances were different, if only you made different decisions in your life? Do you play a certain scenario over and over in your head, thinking how it could have played out differently? Are you always expecting the worst? Do you express your frustration that nothing ever works out for you? Dr Leaf uses an interesting example. She asks whether you are forming a personal identity around, for example, a disease you have. Do you speak of "my condition" or "my heart problem"? Are you overly concerned about what others think of you? Do you worry about what they may say?

Your brain is exceptionally powerful and believes these suggestions. That has a direct impact on your hormonal functions, which in turn, impacts your health. It is interesting that the Bible also refers to the power of words. Proverbs 18:21 of the New Living Translation says: "The tongue can bring death or life; those who love to talk will reap the consequences." We need to watch what we think, but even more what we say.

Dr Leaf highlights that our thoughts have an impact on our nervous, endocrine, immune, intestinal, integumentary, muscular and cardiovascular systems. In the next chapter we will look at these impacts. We will also explore how you can take charge of your thoughts and words.

Detox your environment

The physical environment in which we work and live is so toxic, and the sad part is that we do not realise it. I would like to tell you a bit about my own story. I was diagnosed with Graves Disease in 2015. Graves is an autoimmune disease which attacks the thyroid and causes hyperthyroidism. This means that the thyroid becomes over active. Consequently, my thyroid was enlarged and had multiple nodules growing on it. As medical science tends to run to quick solutions, I was administered radio-active iodine to shrink my thyroid and reduce its activity. Little did I know what the negative effects of radio-active iodine would be on my whole body. I became severely sick overnight. My eyes were swollen, I felt extremely toxic and developed what I thought was a severe allergy. Meanwhile I had chemical sensitivities, not an allergy. I reacted to all chemical fumes.

Without boring you with the details, it took me months of research to get to a point where I managed to get the correct medical advice. I soon realised that a natural approach would have been far more beneficial. One major component of this natural approach was to get rid of all toxins in my diet and immediate environment. Today I am living a healthy and happy life. It took me almost two years to get where I am now. Changing my lifestyle made a huge difference in the first six months. Thereafter the improvement was slow, but steady.

I am amazed at what I learned in that period. Did you know almost everything we use in our households is toxic: from cleaning chemicals, facial creams, bath soaps, plastic containers, to pesticides, etc? In Chapter 6 we will critically review the major toxins in you work and home environments. But more importantly, we will consider healthy alternatives.

Detox your body

Due to the advances in technology and our fast-paced lives where quick fixes and fast food reigns, we are constantly exposed to toxins which mess with our hormone balances. Unfortunately, we can only do so much to contain the toxins we absorb. Fortunately, there is a lot we can do to get rid of the toxin load in our bodies.

Our bodies get rid of toxins mainly though bowel movements, sweat, urine and breathing, which releases carbon dioxide. Thus, the most important detox regimen we can follow is eating well, exercise and deep breathing. In Chapter 6 we go into much more detail on how to detox the body and how to keep our toxin levels low.

Build your house on a Rock

The fourth key is at the centre as depicted in Figure 3. To live at peace with ourselves and others, to be healthy and happy, we need to know why we are here. What is our purpose? Where do we want to go?

If we float aimlessly on a boat at sea with the waves bumping us in all directions, we feel worthless and directionless. We lose all sense of belonging.

In Chapter 7 we will explore the importance of building your house on a Rock. In my case, my faith in God keeps me focused and motivated. Matthew 7:24-27 says: [24]"Everyone then who hears these words of mine and does them will be like a wise man who built his house on the rock. [25] And the rain fell, and the floods came, and the winds blew and beat on that house, but it did not fall, because it had been founded on the rock. [26]And everyone who hears these words of mine and does not do them will be like a foolish man who built his house on the sand. [27]And the rain fell, and the floods came, and the winds blew and beat against that house, and it fell, and great was the fall of it."

It is important to acknowledge that building your house on a rock may mean different things to different people. The bottom line is believing in something bigger than yourself, something or someone that will give you direction and hope and provide you with a safe place to off load your burdens. Whatever your spiritual beliefs, as long as you know what your rock is. Without any further contemplation, let's go through the 4 keys in detail. I can't wait!

Chapter 5 - Detox your Mind

*"If you realised just how powerful your thoughts
are, you would never think a negative thought."*
Peace Pilgrim

As mentioned in the previous chapter, Dr Leaf has done a lot of research on the negative impacts of toxic thoughts on one's body. Just as negative, toxic thoughts negatively impact the body, healthy thoughts have a positive effect. She highlights the following impacts as quoted from her website:

> ➢ "Nervous system – Healthy thoughts literally cause the brain to grow, making you more intelligent. Since the brain is connected via the nervous system to the rest of the body, total health increases.
> ➢ Endocrine system – Healthy thoughts positively affect the hormonal balance, which in turn positively affects the rest of the body's systems. Even fertility can be affected by our thoughts.
> ➢ Immune system – Thoughts affect the functioning of the defenders of the body, the white blood cells. Healthy thoughts lead to robust white blood cells that can fight off infections and even devour cancer cells.
> ➢ Intestinal system – The gut has a 'brain' of its own. A 'gut feeling' is real. Healthy thoughts promote proper digestion and therefore lead to good general health.
> ➢ Integumentary system – This system includes the skin, the largest organ in the body. Healthy thoughts lead to better skin, the body's first line of defence.
> ➢ Muscular system – When your thought life is healthy, you are motivated to exercise. Exercised muscles in turn release substances that increase brain health. This is an example of an upward spiral.

> ➢ Cardiovascular system – Healthy thoughts are involved in proper communication between the heart's mini-brain and the brain in the skull. This promotes well-being, because the heart orchestrates the body's electromagnetic rhythm and harmony. Good thoughts also enhance the vascular system, thus preventing hypertension."

Dr Leaf says in so many words: "There are INTELLECTUAL and MEDICAL reasons to FORGIVE!" A truly profound statement!

Getting rid of emotional pollutants

By now you have clearly seen my passion for getting rid of all sorts of pollutants. Some of the major pollutants in our lives are emotional.

How many of us are entertaining emotional manipulation? Why do we do it? Well, that is simple: to keep the peace. While you are subjected to emotional manipulation or abuse, you are not at peace. Your whole being is crying out. Let me give you an example. I will use illustrative names. Jane had a long-time friend, John, that was emotionally dependent on her. He was always down in the dumps, always going through some sort of crisis. In her effort to keep him up, she pulled herself and her other relationships down. Sounds familiar?

You need to evaluate all your relationships, friends and family included, and decide whether any of them are emotional pollutants. If they are, you need to decide what measures you will put in place to minimise the effect on you. Healthy boundaries are needed.

Healthy boundaries are a necessity, not a nice to have.

One way to establish the impact your relationships have on you is to evaluate your inner circle. The circles below depict all your relationships and where you place people around you. Are they in your inner circle or closer to the outer circle?

Let's do a quick analysis of your inner circle. The people in your inner circle are people close to you. They know you and the challenges you face. They also know the highlights of your life. They know you intimately and you trust them. The middle and outer circles also refer to people close to you, but not as close as the ones in your inner circle. Take a moment to think who you care about the most? Plot the people close to you in terms of where they feature in your circle of friends, from your inner circle to the outer layers.

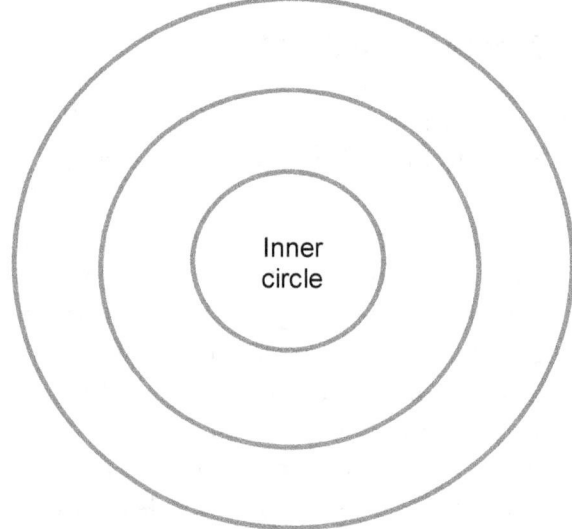

Figure 4: My circle of friends

Now that you have done that, ask yourself: What impact does each individual have on my life? What strategies should I employ in dealing with positive and negative relationships? Take a piece of paper and write down your answers to these questions.

People in your inner circle should have a positive impact on you. The mere fact that they are in your inner circle means that you value their opinions. If they do not build you up, but rather break you down, you may just start believing them. If any one of these individuals has a negative impact on you as a person, you need to ask yourself whether you should retain them in your inner circle. In practice, many people in our inner circles are family members. We can choose our friends, but we can't choose our family. It is always a difficult decision. But if someone is bad for you, and bringing you down, you have one of two choices. One is to remove them from inner circle, and that means maybe from your life as well, or two, you can institute healthy boundaries in that relationship. Many people battle with unhealthy family relationships. The most common example is where marriages are affected by the interference of mothers, fathers, sisters or brothers. Once you are married, the responsibility for managing that marriage lies with you and your spouse. Do not involve your families in any issues you deal with, and do not allow any interference. Place the necessary distance between you and the family members who interfere.

That may mean that you move them to the outer layer of your circle of friends. You may not spend so much time with them as before. You may not answer your phone at all times of day if he/she phones, but give yourself time off. The key is healthy boundaries.

Doreen Virtue said: "Boundaries are healthy, normal and necessary."

Another question when revisiting your circle of friends is: "Do I have too few or too many people in my inner circle?" If you have no people in your inner circle, you will experience a lot of stress because you do not have anybody to share your ups and downs with. The other extreme is having too many people in your inner circle. Maintaining relationships takes time and effort. Having too many people in your inner circle will put pressure on you to find the time and energy to maintain all these relationships.

It is worthwhile at this point to park a moment and think about who we put on our pavilion. We all tend to put the people in our inner circle on our pavilion. Let us use the analogy of a soccer game. If your life is the soccer game, you decided who you put on the pavilion to cheer you on or to 'boo' you off the field. That is the difference between an actual soccer game and your life. You choose!!

More often than not, we get very upset and hurt by the views of those we put on our pavilion. My best advice to you would be to remove them from your pavilion. You are giving them power over you. Only you can remove them!

I think I have made my point. Review the people in your circle of friends and make a conscious decision about any changes you need to make. Do not allow family and friendships to add to your stress. But don't just write people off. Try setting healthy boundaries. Take control of your relationships and manage it.

Manage your romantic relationships

A romantic relationship plays one of two roles in your life. It either builds you up and makes you happy or it induces stress and makes you miserable. You will immediately know whether this section is relevant to your stress levels. Let's look back at your relationships to date and figure out what it is you need or want and then determine what you need to avoid to proactively manage your stress.

Start off by making a list of all the people you have had romantic relationships with. Put them on a continuum, the negative relationships on the left and the constructive ones on the right. Some may be in-between. Note that I do not refer to happy or unhappy. All relationships have their ups and downs. We are looking at relationships that had a good effect on you (constructive), and ones that had a negative effect on you (destructive).

Write down in each relationship what the top 3 things were that you learned from that relationship.

Negative/Destructive   *Constructive*

_____

_____

_____

_____

Once you have added the names and considered the relationships, answer these questions:

1. What do you want in a relationship?
2. What will you avoid in future?
3. More importantly, what will you appreciate in a relationship?
4. What will you bring to a relationship?
5. Given what you've learnt, if married/single, what would you stop doing, what would you do more or less of or start doing to ensure a great relationship?

You can choose what type of relationship you want to have. Be the best you can be in a relationship, and make good choices that will build you up!

Why do we include relationships in detoxing the mind? If your relationships and your thoughts around your relationships are toxic, you need to do something about it. Sometimes there is nothing wrong with our relationships, the problem lies with us and our toxic thoughts. We contemplate nonsense. We create scenarios in our heads which never even happened or never will happen. If this is what you do, stop and think about it. If you are creating silly scenarios in your head of what your partner or spouse is doing or thinking, stop it right now. Take charge of your thoughts and instead of always looking for the negative in all situations, be thankful and appreciative. Express your appreciation towards your partner. Sometimes we should stop thinking about ourselves for a moment and start thinking about others and their needs. If we start to acknowledge and appreciate others, they will mostly return the favour. The bottom line is that we all want to feel appreciated.

I am sure you have all heard about the *5 Love Languages* by Gary Chapman. In his book he describes the five languages as (1) Words of affirmation, (2) Quality time, (3) Receiving gifts, (4) Acts of service and (5) Physical touch. This is a fantastic book that I recommend to everyone in a relationship. So often I have seen men whose love language is acts of service, while the wife's love language is physical touch. The sad outcome of this mismatch is that the man pledges his love by doing things for his wife, which she never appreciates, because she is expecting touch, which he is not giving her.

He starts thinking that she does not appreciate him and does not really care for him, while she thinks he lost all interest in her as her need for physical touch is not fulfilled. She feels unloved. He feels unappreciated. Can you see the irony?! They should both change their thinking and start appreciating what they do for each other.

We need to raise our awareness to the level that we can see things for what they really are. We need to avoid at all cost ruminating on silly thoughts that are not based on fact.

Another major factor impacting our thoughts is unfinished business.

Finish unfinished business

Are you walking around with a load on your shoulders? Is unfinished business from the past haunting you? Is guilt weighing you down? If you want to be strong enough to deal with whatever will still come your way, *you need to let go of the unfinished business of the past*. It literally weighs you down. It wears you out to the extent that you are not able to deal with your daily stress. Let it go!

Unfinished business tends to mull around in our minds and consume our every thought. These thoughts are as toxic as they come.

I know you are probably thinking: "Easy for you to say!" It's not easy, but you have to get it off your shoulders. The best way I know of to deal with unfinished business is to take a piece of paper and write to the person/s with whom you have unfinished business. Write as though you were talking to them. Do not hold anything back. Pretend they are listening to you. If it is someone you are angry with that has hurt you in some way, tell them how you feel. Or it may be someone whom you have wronged and you are carrying the weight of that guilt on your shoulders. Ask them to forgive you. Maybe you need to forgive yourself. Write yourself a letter!

The person you have unfinished business with could have passed away, or he/she could be alive and well. Especially when somebody has passed away, we tend to hold onto these feelings which weigh us down. You will not believe the relief it brings to write these letters. That is, until you do it.

Regardless whether they are alive or have passed on, write a letter from your heart, not holding back. When you are done, hold a little ceremony on your own where you burn these letters and see them go up in smoke. Just make sure that you do it safely. If you are not keen on a fire, tear your letter to pieces and throw it away or bury it. It's amazing what an impact such symbolic ceremonies have.

If the person is still alive and you are able to work things out with him/her in person, even better. Forgiveness will set you free. Do not wait with this exercise. Get a piece of paper and start writing this minute.

Manage yourself

The question in your mind right now could be: where do I start? The answer is cognitive behaviour therapy. **Cognitive behaviour therapy (CBT) is a talk therapy that can help you manage your problems by changing the way you think and behave. It is most commonly used to treat anxiety and depression, but can be useful for other mental and physical health problems.** Let's make CBT practical.

Managing yourself is step 1 on your road to sustainable high performance. Managing yourself proactively can greatly enhance the way you deal with stress. By now you know whether you are more of a Type A or Type B personality. Especially if you are a Type A personality, you need to conscientiously manage your personality to reduce your negative stress levels.

The first step is to create an awareness of your emotions, your thoughts and your behaviour.

Today you need to take charge of your thoughts, your emotions and your behaviour. In the model below you can clearly see how your emotions, thoughts and behaviour interact and influence one another on a continuous basis. If you feel angry at someone, your thoughts tend to go into a negative spiral, and if you tend to be an expressive person, your behaviour would show it. At the same time, if you feel happy about something, you will experience more happy thoughts and may even dance in delight to demonstrate your happiness through your behaviour.

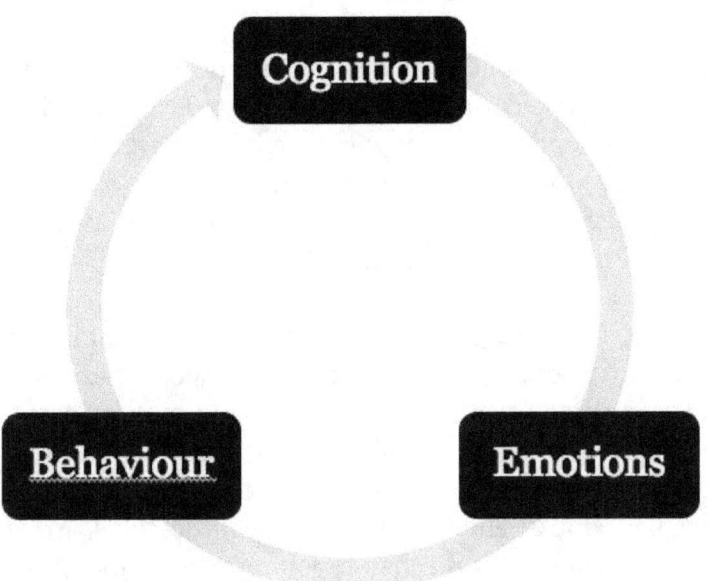

Figure 5: The Self-Management Cycle

The theory is that if you can take charge of your thoughts, you can directly impact your emotions and your behaviour.

We tend to think that it always starts with an emotion. Reality is that the cycle could start with an emotion, a thought or behaviour. And the one influences the other.

Let explore a real example. A few years ago I woke up one morning feeling miserable. You know the feeling when everything in your life is just not going to plan. The last thing I felt like was getting out of bed and starting work on my current project. Being self-employed and having a home office did not help. It meant if I wanted to, I could just turn around, pull the pillow over my head and continue sleeping. That is exactly how I felt. But, knowing the psychology behind it, I knew that if I got up and put myself in an environment that I liked, that my emotions and my thinking would adapt accordingly. I got up (reluctantly), packed my laptop and went to the botanical gardens – my favourite get-away. I went and sat in the tea garden, not far from the waterfall. I unpacked my laptop and started working in the picturesque environment. The birds were singing, the water from the fall crashing, I could smell the flowers and the clean air, and feel the soft breeze on my skin. Within 20 minutes I felt like a different person. I was working with dedication and feeling at peace.

What happened? I woke up with a certain emotion, and started thinking (cognition) about it, which resulted in a specific behaviour. My instinctive behaviour was to stay in bed and sulk. Instead I decided to change my behaviour and go to the park, which in turn changed both my emotions and cognitive thinking. The bottom-line is when feeling bad; don't behave according to your feelings. You can take charge of your behaviour and change your emotions and thinking accordingly.

You can use the model in any direction. Let me give you another example. Julie was harassed by her previous boss. He used to look over her shoulder at what she was doing on her computer, breathing down her neck. She had some very bad memories. After a few incidents, she resigned and changed jobs. At her new job, her manager one day stormed into her office, urgently looking for information. He ran up to her and looked over her shoulder (coming very close to her, not knowing what happened to her in the past). Before he could express what he wanted, she flew up and ran out of her office. He just stood there wondering what happened.

In this example, Julie had a particular frame of reference. When her new boss stormed into her office and came close to her, she thought (cognition) that he was up to no good. That immediately created fear (emotion) within her and she ran out of her office (behaviour). Through an awareness of her paradigm (fear of harassment by a boss), she could have influenced her thinking when he approached her. She could have told herself immediately that this was not the same person who harassed her before. She could have asked him what he wanted and told him that she was not comfortable with him storming into her office without warning. Once she had established why he had approached her, she would automatically have felt more comfortable and would not have fled. You can now see that by being aware of your thoughts (cognition), you can change them, which in turn will affect your emotions and your behaviour. You can use this model from any angle.

Let's explore one last example. People suffering from depression fit into two main categories; those who have a chemical imbalance in the brain that causes the depression and those who have mastered the art of negative self-talk. If you fit into the first category, you need medical help. If you fit into the second, you can apply these principles with great success. Positive self-talk is a very powerful tool in maintaining a healthy emotional state, and consequently a healthy physical state. In the next section on psychoneuroimmunology we will explore this link.

Be conscious of your thoughts, your emotions and your behaviour and at all times be in control of it.

You will only master this principle with practice. It starts with awareness, followed by practice.

This experience is further enhanced by speaking to yourself out loud. If you hear yourself, chances are increased that you would listen and respond.

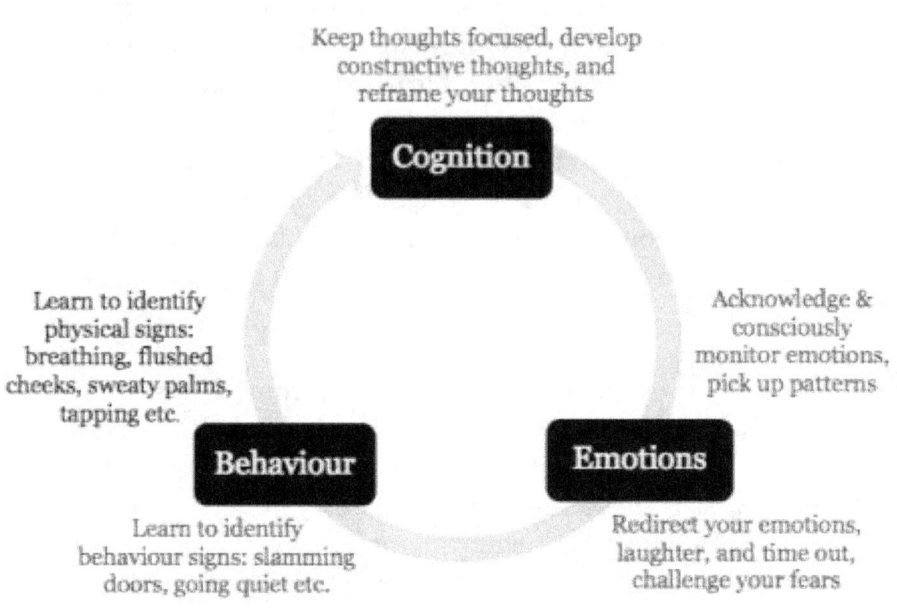

Figure 6: Managing Yourself Using the Self-Management Cycle

In summary, keep your thoughts focused. Always be aware of what you are thinking, because it is affecting you in more ways than you realise. When you pick up on a negative or toxic thought pattern, break it. Consciously change it into constructive thoughts. Also, be aware of your emotions. Acknowledge them. Redirect them by talking to a good friend, laughing, taking time out, doing gardening, and yes, challenging your fears. You can see that changing your behaviour has a profound impact on your emotions. Just as you need to improve your awareness of your emotions and thoughts, you also need to be more aware of your behaviour and physical symptoms – your breathing, your cheeks flushing or your palms sweating. If you pick up on it, immediately assess your thoughts and emotions, and most of all, take charge! Do something about it.

Let's for a moment consider the cycle of loss. In no particular sequence, after we have lost something or someone, we experience the following: denial, depression, anger, grief and acceptance. When losing someone or something dear to us, we normally first tend to go into denial. We do not want to believe what has happened to us. It's not possible. Maybe it is just a bad dream and I will wake up from it. We then wake up one morning and denial is gone, and we realise what we've lost. Then we either go into depression, anger or grief. When we are depressed, we withdraw from people and want to pull the blanket over our heads in the morning and not get up. At some point, we are angry at anyone we can blame for what has been taken away from us. We get angry with ourselves, angry with God and angry with any person we can link to our loss. Anger is often a very good coping mechanism to hide our real feelings of pain, sadness and disappointment. Anger normally precedes grief. Grief is a critical phase in the cycle. It allows us to feel the pain of losing someone. Once you have gone through all of these phases, however quickly or slowly, you can achieve acceptance. At this point you can make peace with what has happened to you. We often go back to a certain stage, but then tend to stay there for a shorter time before we move on. The Self-Management Cycle can help you prevent getting stuck in the depression phase, which often happens.

The question now remains: how do we apply these principles in managing our personalities? I am a Type A personality. I am thus always very aware of the fact that I want things done well and as quickly as possible (according to my standards). In asking a less experienced person to assist me with a job, I am constantly aware that I may expect the same level of delivery as I would have given. My behaviour tends to show signs of impatience. I would tap, my voice would become cold and directive, my thoughts would run off thinking: "What is she doing? Does she even know what she is doing?" You can see, in my own mind I take this 'thing' and I run with it. The more I do that, the greater my anger, frustration and dissatisfaction. By increasing my awareness of my emotions, behaviour and thoughts, I have learned to manage my reactions. I consciously change my thoughts to: "She is new and inexperienced. She has not been around the block a few times. I wonder how I can help her. Maybe I can do something to guide her to get it right." Immediately I don't get anxious any more. I am more tolerant and don't display impatient behaviour.

It may sound easy. Trust me, it is not. It takes a lot of practice and effort from your side. You need to work at it. Sometimes you need to fake it, like I did the day I went to the botanical gardens. I did not feel like it, but I forced myself to change my behaviour. It worked! Your journey starts now...

Psychoneuroimmunology

Psychoneuroimmunology is the scientific study of the link between emotions, the nervous system and the immune function. Your thoughts, moods, emotions and belief systems impact your health. It has been scientifically proven that positive and negative mind-states result in chemical reactions in the body, which can either compromise or enhance your immune function. Positive thoughts and attitudes discharge chemicals in the brain that build your immune system.

Examples include flexibility (the willingness to adapt to circumstances), acknowledgement that stress is positive as long as you feel in control, expression of your emotions and assertiveness in expressing yourself.

On the other hand, a negative state of mind compromises your immune system. Examples of these are suppressed emotions, feelings of helplessness and being out of control, knowing something is wrong and not taking action to rectify it, unresolved feelings of guilt, fear or failure and unfinished business. My guess is that you can associate yourself with at least two of these, if not more.

Scientific studies on laughing have shown a tremendous positive impact on the health of research subjects.

Another interesting fact is that your pursuit of goals related to living a meaningful life also boosts your immune system.

Having a purpose in life and pursuing it vigorously makes you happy. The moral of the story is: be aware (conscious) of your thoughts, which will put you in a position to manage them. As far as possible, always attempt to turn negative thoughts and emotions into positive ones. It starts with awareness of your thoughts, followed by a conscious rethink of your thoughts, which will impact your emotions. Only you can choose whether you influence them positively or negatively.

The Self-Management Cycle clearly shows how your emotions, behaviour and thoughts are interlinked, while Psychoneuro-immunology adds to that by emphasising the fact that your thoughts and emotions have an impact on your health. Therefore, it is imperative that you increase your awareness of your thoughts and emotions and manage these actively to stay positive at all times.

So what can you do? You need to start practising positive self-talk. When you don't feel like doing something, be firm and encourage yourself to do it.

If you feel like the whole world has turned against you, focus on all the positives in your life. Think about what you have and be thankful for all your blessings.

Inevitably this discussion takes us to the topic of depression. More often than not our feelings of depression originate from someone else that is close to us, who might be dealing with their own problems. You can be there for them, but they need to take responsibility for their own lives, and you for yours. *Expose yourself to positive people.* You know who makes you smile and who motivates you. Spend more time with those people!

Fight Fear

The root of all worry (stress) is fear. They say: "Don't worry, be happy". To be in that happy state, you need to resist and fight fear with all you have. In our beautiful country South Africa, we walk around with the fear of being robbed, being high-jacked, our family leaving the country, keeping our jobs, and so many more. Fear is the direct opposite of faith. You need to have faith that all will be well.

You need to believe that nothing bad will happen to you. By believing, then planning, followed by action, you can destroy fear.

Let's take an example. If you fear that your family will leave the country, you are likely to be unhappy most of the time. You will feel a mixture of sadness, fear, anger and frustration. If your family member wants to leave the country, you can't prevent them from doing so. You need to plan. Do you want to go as well? If yes, then get the ball rolling. Find out which country is best suited for your family on a personal level and where work opportunities are optimal. If you want to stay, enjoy every second with your family today. Use the time you have left. Furthermore, you can explore technologies to help you communicate with your family, such as webcam. Take action to create an environment in which you will be able to maintain contact at a distance.

What really helps when it comes to managing fear is to ask yourself: "What is the worst that can happen?" Let's use an example. If you fear retrenchment, the worst that can happen is that you will get retrenched. You will, however, get a severance package. At worst you will need to find another job, start your own business or take early retirement.

Through planning, followed by action on your side, you take responsibility and make sure your fears don't paralyse you.

In summary on thoughts

If you have never been aware of what you were thinking and saying before, now is the time to raise your awareness, take charge of your thoughts, and start thinking and speaking constructive, uplifting messages.

I know too many people who are caught up in a spiral of negative thoughts. It is time to let go of these toxic thoughts. Take charge and change your life!

Chapter 6 - Detox your Environment

"Your body is ground zero in the battle of pollution." Andy Igrejas

In the previous chapter, we looked at the soft stuff which is typically the hard stuff. In this chapter, we will look at your physical environment. Making changes to your physical environment is much easier and can reap great benefits!

Let's consider some examples. Being stuck in traffic every day and being exposed to exhaust fumes is a major stressor. Living in crowded areas is another stressor for many South Africans, especially those living in townships. A vast number of people live in townhouses. If you drive through the major cities in South Africa, much of what you see are the rooftops of houses, one after another. To address the security issue in South Africa, property developers have focused on the development of cluster homes and townhouses. Thinking back to my youth, I was brought up in a big house in Pretoria, with a huge garden. Since I have left home, I have not experienced such openness anywhere I stayed.

You need to take a critical look at your environment and clearly define your environmental stressors.

Only once I was diagnosed with Graves Disease did I realise the importance of managing my environmental pollutants. I remember telling my endocrinologist that I wake up feeling intoxicated. That is exactly what happened! As soon as I started to detox my environment, my health improved immediately.

I would like to walk you through your house and make you aware of toxins you did not realise existed up to now. Let's consider a few.

Cleaning chemicals

Cleaning chemicals are a major culprit. Some of the basic ingredients in dish washing liquid and washing detergent include surfactants, preservatives, fragrance, dyes and anti-bacterial ingredients (either active or inactive). They also contain phthalates (synthetic fragrance) which are hormone-disrupting chemicals. These are toxic to the body and can cause allergic reactions, skin irritations and respiratory issues. A good reference you can use is the website https://gimmethegoodstuff.org/. Throughout this chapter I will reference many articles which you can read if you are interested. I prefer to keep the book short and concise, but I know some of you may want to learn more.

Apart from detergents and dish washing liquid, there are toxic chemicals in a host of other household cleaning products, such as ammonia, toilet cleaners, bathroom cleaners, window cleaners, bleach and so forth.

I will refrain from going into detail of what each of these chemicals is capable of. I would like to help you make better decisions when buying dish washing liquid, however. You should look for the following:

➤ Plant-based surfactants (or just plain soap)
➤ Dye-free
➤ 1,4 Dioxane-free
➤ Phthalate-free
➤ Petrochemical-free
➤ Glycol-free
➤ Phosphate-free
➤ Caustic-free

There are many organic, toxin-free alternatives on the market. If you search the internet, you will also find many natural soap recipes which you can try.

Indoor air contamination

Indoor air contamination comes from various sources, such as toxins trapped in carpets, flame retardant treatments in your upholstery and paint on walls. Volatile organic compounds (VOCs), which are airborne chemicals implicated in a range of ill health effects, should be limited in your home. Ideally speaking we should replace our sofas and mattresses with products that are made from flame retardant material. This is likely to be a challenge for most of us. If you can, replace all composite wood that go by names such as pressed wood, compressed wood, plywood, particle board, or medium density fibreboard (MDF). These all omit VOCs. Replace furniture with 100% solid wood if possible.

Unfortunately, wood needs furniture polish, which can be even more toxic. Furniture polish contains hydrocarbons (waxes, oils, organic solvents), which can cause a whole range of symptoms. A product that I have grown to love is coconut oil. It is a fantastic alternative to furniture polish. You can use very little and will be surprised how much it nourishes your furniture.

You can also invest in a good quality vacuum cleaner (a HEPA-sealed model), which ensures that dust and toxins stay sealed inside the filter. It is better to vacuum and wet mop than to sweep.

Another option is to get rid of your carpets and replace them with tiles.

And finally, if you can, repaint your home with non-toxic paints. Visit your local paint dealer and enquire about eco paints.

BPA

Bisphenol A, also known as BPA, is an industrial chemical that is used in the manufacture of certain plastics and resins. It is used in containers that store food and beverages. It is also used to coat the inside of metal products, such as food cans, bottle tops, plastic containers and water supply lines.

Exposure to BPA is a concern because of its possible health effects on the brain, behaviour and prostate glands of foetuses, infants and children.

According to The Food and Drug Administration (FDA) as quoted by Bauer on the Mayo Clinic website, BPA is safe at the very low levels that occur in some foods.

Bauer says that the FDA is, however, continuing its review of BPA, including supporting ongoing research. In the meantime, if you're concerned about BPA, you can take these steps to reduce your exposure:

> ➢ Use BPA-free products
> ➢ Reduce your use of canned foods since most cans are lined with BPA-containing resin
> ➢ Avoid heat. The National Institute of Environmental Health Sciences, a part of the National Institutes of Health, advises against microwaving polycarbonate plastics or putting them in the dishwasher, because the plastic may break down over time and allow BPA to leach into foods. The same goes for leaving plastic water bottles in cars that are exposed to the sun. Rather use a glass bottle.
> ➢ Use alternatives, such as glass, porcelain or stainless steel containers for hot foods and liquids, instead of plastic containers.

Tap water

Dr Edward Group (2016) published a very enlightening article on the 12 toxins in tap water (http://www.globalhealingcenter.com/natural-health/12-toxins-in-your-drinking-water/). Most of these toxins cannot even be pronounced. I would like to discuss four of these: fluoride, chlorine, lead and mercury. If you are interested in the rest, use the link above.

Fluoride is a neurotoxin and an endocrine disruptor. It can harm the thyroid gland and calcify the pineal gland. Chlorine is a reactive chemical that bonds with water, including the water in your gut, to produce poisonous hydrochloric acid. Chlorine exposure can cause respiratory problems and damage cells. Lead is toxic to almost every organ. Mercury is extremely toxic and can cause multiple illnesses.

I am sure you must be thinking that this cannot be true and that the amounts must be so low that it will not have an effect. Something I have realised over the last few years is that the compounding effect of the multiple toxins we are exposed to can severely affect our health. I have taken multiple measures to reduce the toxin load I am exposed to. Believe me, I am reaping the benefit!

Boiling water certainly helps as it kills bacteria. Unfortunately, it does not remove toxins like fluoride. The best solution is to change to filtered water. Filtering clears out many safety concerns like bacteria, heavy metals and pesticides. You can either buy your water from a recognised water supplier or fit your kitchen with a high-quality water filter. Do note that some water filters do not remove fluoride.

One more option may be to harvest rain water.

Beauty products

This is a very sensitive subject. When I started removing toxins from my immediate environment, I soon learned that my perfume had the worst effect on my health. The moment I stopped using my perfume, my health improved.

Perfume contains phthalates and fragrances which are endocrine disrupters. To protect trade secrets, perfume manufacturers are allowed to withhold fragrance ingredients, so consumers can't rely on labels to know what hazards may lurk inside that bottle of perfume.

Fortunately, we have some healthy alternatives available at leading pharmacies and health shops. I prefer making my own using essential oils. I am so sensitive to perfumes that if I sit in church next to someone wearing heavy perfume, my head starts pounding, I itch and my eyes start to swell. I would go so far to say that changing my perfume and cleaning chemicals to natural alternatives had the biggest positive impact on my health.

Just as perfume is loaded with toxic fragrances which manufacturers do not have to divulge, so are bath soaps and creams, facial creams and so forth. I replaced all my facial products with rooibos extract or aloe based products which have no toxic ingredients.

Another unsuspected culprit is cosmetics. An excellent website to visit is www.safecosmetics.org. This website started a campaign for safe cosmetics. They discuss all the cosmetic ingredients that should raise your eyebrows. They highlight toxic ingredients in products such as sun screen, make-up, creams, shampoos and conditioners, hairspray, personal care products, soaps, detergents, toothpastes and deodorants, to mention but a few. It is worth it to invest in toxic free, green cosmetic products. To my surprise these healthy, non-toxic alternatives are fairly priced.

At this point I would like to discuss my favourite alternative, namely coconut oil.

Dr Axe wrote an article where he outlines 77 uses of coconut oil. To visit his web page, go to https://draxe.com/coconut-oil-uses/.

I regularly use coconut oil for the following:
> Furniture polish
> Body lotion
> Hair mask/conditioner
> Homemade toothpaste, mixed with bicarbonate of soda to form a paste
> Natural deodorant – mix a little bicarbonate of soda and essential oils
> Sunscreen
> Insect repellent: mix a tablespoon of coconut oil with a couple of drops of peppermint, rosemary, and tea tree oil to repel flies and mosquitoes.

Seeing that I mentioned toothpaste in the list above, it is worthwhile to mention that it is loaded with fluoride that interferes with your thyroid function.

To date I have replaced all my facial products, body creams, shower gels, hair products, make-up, nail polish, deodorants and perfumes with natural products. Some I buy from my local pharmacy, some from health shops and some I make at home. The impact on my health has been incredible. If you battle with constant allergies or asthma, I highly recommend that you try detoxing your environment.

Laundry detergents

Earlier I mentioned the toxicity in laundry detergents and fabric softeners. They also contain hormone disrupting fragrances. A great alternative is bicarbonate of soda, better known as baking soda. You will be surprised, you won't even need softener.

Air fresheners

Air fresheners are loaded with VOCs that are highly toxic. They also contain phthalates which were mentioned earlier. These are hormone-disrupting chemicals. Sarah Corriher published a very interesting article on this subject. You can go to http://healthwyze.org/reports/184-how-air-fresheners-are-killing-you to read more about it.

There are multiple non-toxic alternatives on the market which use a blend of essential oils. They smell fresh and do not harm your body. Do yourself a favour and visit your local health shop.

Insecticides and pesticides

We all know that household insecticides and pesticides should be toxic. They are designed to get rid of pests. Unfortunately, they are just as toxic to humans.

Derek Markham (2016) shares some very interesting homemade insecticide recipes in this article http://www.treehugger.com/lawn-garden/8-natural-homemade-insecticides-save-your-garden-without-killing-earth.html.

There are products on the market which are bio-degradable and less toxic. They are more expensive, but effective. And most importantly, they do not lead to respiratory illnesses.

Exhaust fumes

Exposure to exhaust fumes is inevitable. Most of us are stuck in traffic on a daily basis.

I have developed the habit of closing my air vents when in dense traffic. It at least helps to keep some of the toxins out. Another strategy is to change your route to work to one that carries less traffic. Or if you can, work flexi-hours and avoid heavy traffic all together.

Fire place smoke

We all love the feeling of a fire place. It creates a cosy and warm atmosphere. The Cleveland Clinic published an article on their website to highlight the dangers of fire place smoke https://health.clevelandclinic.org/2014/12/that-cozy-fire-could-be-hazardous-to-your-health/.

The best solution is to limit your exposure by installing a fire place with a door which closes tightly and doesn't emit smoke into the house.

Non-stick pots and pans

I am sure you love non-stick pans as much as I do. Unfortunately, they are covered with a synthetic polymer which is toxic. In this article, http://www.ewg.org/research/healthy-home-tips/tip-6-skip-non-stick-avoid-dangers-teflon, the Environmental Working Group (EWG) unpacks the dangers of using non-stick pans. They indicate that when heated, it releases toxic fumes that may kill pet birds and cause people to develop flu-like symptoms.

Safer options are stainless steel, ceramic or cast iron pots and pans. One way to limit your risk with a non-stick pan is to cook your food over low temperatures.

Ergonomics

Ergonomics refer to the way your physical environment is set up. You are now probably wondering what that has to do with stress management.

To practice a proactive stress management philosophy, you need to make sure that your physical living and work environment is set up to produce the least amount of stress to your body.

Consideration should be given to the lighting where you live and work, the height of your office chair, the positioning of your phone and the direction of your computer screen relative to the window in your office. As for the height of your seat, it is optimal once your elbows are at a 90-degree angle with the desk. That way you remove pressure from your neck. If you suffer from chronic neck stiffness, your first step should be to review the height of your seat relative to your desk.

If you are left-handed, it is best to position your phone on the right-hand side of your computer and the opposite if you are right-handed.

Another potentially major stressor to your body is the way your seat is positioned in your car, your office and in front of the television. You should always sit as upright as possible with support to your lower back. A few years ago I suffered from chronic back ache. I tried everything to get rid of it. I then looked for the root cause of my back ache. I always try to identify the cause, so that I can address the problem at its root and not treat the symptoms. I analysed when my back ache started. I soon realised it started just when I bought my new car. What a light bulb moment! Yes, my new car seat wasn't positioned correctly. I travel a lot, and the seat positioning put so much strain on my back that I could barely handle it. Once I found the correct position of the seat, I still had to do a bit of physiotherapy to get rid of the spasm, but the chronic backache was something of the past. If you spend a lot of time in your car, ensure your seat is positioned such that it supports your back, rather than putting strain on it.

Most living room chairs don't provide proper support to the lower back, which can lead to chronic lower back ache. If you do suffer from lower back pain, take a look at the chairs you use and determine whether it gives you the support you need.

One last example I need to mention is the exercise equipment you use. Due to crime levels in South Africa, we tend to try and spend some time in the gym, or even set up home gyms. Gym equipment is designed such that you can adapt it to the length or built of the person using the equipment. I have found that when I do go to the gym, I am often too lazy to adjust the equipment to my height. Inevitably it then puts strain on me rather than doing any good. Rather adjust the equipment to fit your body, otherwise your effort to manage your stress via exercise becomes one of your stressors.

These are a few examples just to make you aware of the impact of poor or good ergonomics on your body.

Electronic equipment

Electronic devices are a complex mixture of several hundred components. A mobile phone, for example, contains 500 to 1000 components. Many of these contain toxic heavy metals such as lead, mercury, cadmium and beryllium, as well as hazardous chemicals, such as brominated flame retardants. Polluting polyvinyl chloride (PVC) plastic is also frequently used.

Two commonly used items that affect us without us necessarily knowing it are cell phones and television remote controls. The electromagnetic radiation is harmful.

David Morehouse unpacks research on the topic in this article http://www.bibliotecapleyades.net/scalar_tech/esp_scalartech27.htm and provides some tips on how to reduce your exposure.

He suggests the following:

> Use a high quality headset and use it all the time. Avoid holding a phone up to your head.
> The lower your battery level on the phone, the harder the phone works to interrogate the microwave towers it communicates with. This results in more electromagnetic radiation being produced. Therefore, it is best to keep your phone charged and rather use a landline when your cell phone battery is low.
> Signal strength is also a factor. If the signal strength is low, your cell phone must pump out more radiation, again increasing its detrimental effect. Try not to use the phone unless the signal strength is near 100% or use a landline.
> If you carry your phone in your pants pocket, purchase a shielding device that will keep it from radiating your private parts.
> Avoid using your cell phone in a car as the shielding and tinting on newer automobiles cause the electromagnetic waves to bounce back and forth inside the vehicle, exposing you and your passengers to increased levels of radiation.

When you go to bed, make sure not to leave your cell phone, remote control, computer or tablet next to your bed.

Cigarettes

At the risk of boring you, I do not want to go into all the negatives of smoking and secondary smoke. Go ahead and read this article http://www.heart.org/HEARTORG/HealthyLiving/QuitSmoking/QuittingSmoking/Smoking-Do-you-really-know-the-risks_UCM_322718_Article.jsp#.WG93oXdhodU if you are interested. If you do not want to quit for yourself, do it for those around you.

Painkillers

One of my pet hobbies is making people aware of the toxic nature of painkillers. Prolonged use of painkillers, due to the toxins they contain, can cause headaches. In this very interesting article, http://realhealthtalk.com/pain_I_haven't_got_time_for_the_pain_reliever.html, Craig Stellpflug discusses the risks of using painkillers and suggests natural alternatives. What I found very interesting about the article is that he suggests avoiding gluten, as it causes inflammation and therefore induces pain. Just be aware that while you try to get off painkillers, you are likely to experience detox symptoms, which could result in headaches. But do know that it is worth it.

There are many natural alternatives for pain, such as turmeric, Ogema, ginger and capsaicin, which is found in cayenne pepper.

In summary on toxins in your environment

Hopefully by now you will appreciate the magnitude of toxins and strains we are unknowingly exposed to.

Nobody will convince me that the cumulative effect of all these toxins will not affect us. I am living proof.

I followed a step-by-step process, replacing one toxin at a time with natural alternatives. It is amazing how much better I feel. I used to be fatigued and my body aching all the time. This was due to inflammation in my muscles, because of high toxicity levels. If you are constantly tired and in pain, it is worth it to give it a try!

Toxic fumes are detrimental to your health. People often get cold and flu symptoms after exposure to toxic fumes, not realising that the fumes are affecting their lungs. If you want to protect your body, and be proactive in terms of ensuring long-term health, you need to be aware of what you expose yourself to. The message throughout this book is that if you do not look after yourself; your body won't be able to cope with life's daily and inevitable stressors.

The exciting news is that the contrary is also true. Limit the toxins you are exposed to and build a body that is strong enough to endure a lot!

Chapter 7 - Detox your Body

"Most people have no idea how good their body is designed to feel." Kevin Trudeau

As we have seen in Chapter 6, we have control over what we put into our bodies. So it is better to avoid the toxins, rather than trying to get rid of them afterwards.

Eat Healthy

One of the best ways to proactively manage (lessen) the effects of stress on your body, is through healthy eating habits.

There are many schools of thought on healthy eating, but most of them have some elements in common. The following general healthy eating guidelines will greatly contribute to healthy living.

It is important to remember that all the recommendations below are general guidelines. They do not take into account any specific medical condition that you may have. Always consult your medical practitioner or a nutritionist on what you should and should not eat if you have a medical condition.

Limit your sugar intake

Refined sugar is one of the greatest evils of our time. Both granulated refined sugar and high fructose corn syrup go through a refining process. They are called "empty calories" because they have no nutritional value. Yet they are addictive and rob your body of energy and health. According to Dr Axe, side-effects of refined sugars include diabetes, tooth decay, obesity, heart disease, certain types of cancer and even poor cognitive functioning. He states that fructose is a simple sugar that is rapidly metabolised by the liver, causing a "sugar high." This quick-acting sugar is believed to lead to increased storage of fat in the liver, resulting in non-alcoholic fatty liver disease, digestive upset and atherosclerosis.

But what about artificial sweeteners? According to Dr Axe, the list of medical conditions linked to aspartame consumption is extensive and includes:

- anxiety
- depression
- short-term memory loss
- multiple sclerosis
- fibromyalgia
- hearing loss
- weight gain
- fatigue
- brain tumours

Although these illnesses may not all be caused directly by aspartame consumption, it may exacerbate the symptoms. Aspartame can also increase the risk of strokes and cancer. Overall, limit or eliminate consumption of aspartame.

Instead of using aspartame as a sweetener, choose raw local honey or natural stevia, which is much easier to digest and process and benefits your health.

To have a strong immune system that functions effectively, it is best to reduce your sugar intake. Fruit contains fructose. Fruit that contain high levels of fructose include lychees, figs, mangos, cherries, dates, raisins and grapes. Fruits with low sugar content are lemons, limes, apricots, cranberries, kiwi fruits, raspberries, oranges and pears. When eating fruit with high sugar content, it is best to limit your intake. Do not stop eating fruit as it is good for you, but be aware of your sugar intake.

Once you start removing sugar from your diet, you will immediately feel the impact on your body. Your energy levels will rise significantly and will be far more stable. Consider honey and stevia as sugar alternatives, but use it in moderation.

Avoid gluten

Gluten is a family of proteins found in grains like wheat and rye. Some people can tolerate gluten, but those with gluten intolerance and autoimmune diseases battle with gluten. The most common symptoms of gluten intolerance are bloating, belly pain and discomfort, diarrhoea, feeling unwell, aches and tiredness.

If you experience any of these symptoms, it is worthwhile cutting gluten from your diet for two or three weeks and observe the effect. You won't even have to do tests to confirm your gluten intolerance. You will feel the difference. But do not go half way, go all the way.

Keep your blood sugar balanced

One of our worst habits is to get so focused on work that we forget to eat. We may have breakfast before we go to work, but once we get there, we become so engaged with issues at hand, that we only realise when we get home at night that we had nothing to eat during the day. Meanwhile, we consume cup of coffee after cup of coffee to keep up our energy levels.

The energy dips we experience are caused by drops and spikes in our blood sugar levels.

So, what can we do?

- ➢ Whenever we eat a carbohydrate, it should be accompanied by a quality source of fat such as coconut oil, avocado or butter. Fat slows down the absorption of glucose into the bloodstream and prevents sugar highs and sugar crashes.
- ➢ Eat breakfast and include a protein in your breakfast. If we skip breakfast, the body increases production of stress hormones and starts to break down muscle to use for energy. It's very stressful on the body and wreaks havoc with the blood sugar balance for the rest of the day. If you do not enjoy eating an egg for breakfast, you can have a plain yogurt smoothie with ground flaxseed and berries.
- ➢ Eat nuts as a snack, but avoid too many peanuts. I started eating three Brazilian nuts a day to help with my selenium intake (a potent antioxidant). I found this had an amazing impact on balancing my blood sugar.
- ➢ A good night's sleep also contributes to a balanced blood sugar level.
- ➢ Balance you blood sugar by reducing sugar and stimulants such as coffee, fizzy drinks, and chocolates!

Stick with good carbs

The debate around carbohydrates will be a never ending one. From experience I know that my body needs carbohydrates. Instead of obtaining carbohydrates from grains, rather go for healthy ones from fresh fruits and root vegetables. These carbohydrates do not perpetuate inflammation or intestinal damage like grains do. Enjoy fresh fruit in season, as well as a variety of frozen fruit. Sweet potatoes, carrots, beets and other root vegetables provide a nutrient-rich source of healthy carbohydrates. Remember to balance blood sugar, enjoy fruit and roots in the presence of healthy fats and protein.

Avoid the bad carbohydrates such as refined grains, sugary cereals, sugary fizzy drinks, cookies and sweets.

I emphasise once again that these suggestions do not take into account specific health conditions. If you have any medical condition, contact your doctor before changing your diet.

Stick with organic whole foods

Another evil of our time is processed foods. Almost everything we have in our kitchen is processed. If it contains any ingredients which you can barely pronounce, chances are almost 100% that it is processed. Avoid all processed food. They are stripped of nutrients. The more organic you can eat the better. Anything you buy that is pre-prepared is also likely to be processed.

Whole foods have not been processed or refined and is free from additives or other artificial substances. We battle to digest processed foods properly. Whole foods, on the other hand, digest far better.

Most of the vegetables and fruit we buy in super markets are coated in pesticides. Similarly, the meat we buy is loaded with hormones. Stick to organic food as far as possible. I started my own vegetable garden. I cannot explain how incredibly nice it is to walk into the garden and harvest fresh salad and vegetables. I know my garden is organic and pesticide free!

Reduce fried foods and foods high in saturated fat. In other words, avoid junk food. Fortunately, most junk food outlets now also sell salads or other healthy alternatives.

Rather eat lean meat, fish and chicken that are not processed. If prepared well with some tasty seasoning, you will be pleasantly surprised what you can dish up. If possible, stick to organic meats which are not full of hormones.

Limit your dairy intake

Dr Hyman quotes research done by Dr Willet which indicates that about 75% of the world's population is genetically unable to properly digest milk and other dairy products — a problem called lactose intolerance. He states that most humans naturally stop producing significant amounts of lactase, which is the enzyme needed to properly metabolise lactose (the sugar in milk), sometime between the ages of two and five. Most mammals stop producing the enzymes needed to properly digest and metabolise milk after they have been weaned.

Our bodies weren't made to digest milk on a regular basis. Instead, most scientists agree that it's better for us to get calcium, potassium, protein, and fats from other food sources, like whole plant foods (vegetables, fruit, beans, whole grains, nuts and seeds).

If you want to learn more about why milk is not necessarily good for you, take a look at this article: http://nutritionstudies.org/12-frightening-facts-milk/.

Stop toxifying your body

Reduce oxidants and increase antioxidants. This links up with the section on detoxing your environment. We have to think twice about drinking alcohol, smoking or drinking excessive amounts of coffee, to mention but a few examples. Some of us have sugar addictions and can't go a day without a chocolate. These are all oxidants which toxify our bodies.

Go for Himalayan salt

An article by the American Heart Association (2015) states that too much sodium (salt) in your system results in your body retaining water. This puts an extra burden on the heart and blood vessels. In some people this may lead to high blood pressure. Having less sodium in your diet may help you lower or avoid high blood pressure. People with high blood pressure are more likely to develop heart disease or have a stroke.

Most of the sodium in our diet comes from adding it when food is prepared and from processed foods. Pay attention to food labels, because they indicate the amount of sodium in the product.

What is the alternative? Herbs and certain spices have amazing health benefits. When buying spices, look at the ingredients and avoid those that contain monosodium glutamate (MSG), a flavour enhancer. Making a decision to avoid MSG in your diet as much as possible is a wise choice. It does take a bit more planning and time in the kitchen to prepare food at home, using fresh, locally grown ingredients. Knowing that your food is pure and free of toxic additives, like MSG, will make it well worth it.

Try flavouring your food with herbs. Another great option is Himalayan salt. It is said to be the purest salt on earth. Himalayan salt is 85% sodium chloride, and the remainder contains 80+ minerals. These minerals can help your body balance your PH, regulate water content, remove toxins, help absorb nutrients, prevent muscle cramping, create balance and more. It is known for its pure taste and unique pinkish colour.

Do not eat before you go to bed

Night time eating can interfere with sleep, weight control and overall health. Our bodies aren't designed to eat a big meal and collapse on the couch or the bed afterwards. Sitting upright helps digest our food. It lets gravity do the work of keeping the contents of our stomach down. In people with heartburn, lying down can cause the acid in the stomach to leak out into the oesophagus, causing reflux. As the stomach takes about three hours to be emptied, waiting at least that long before lying down or sleeping is a good idea.

Drink water

Drink at least six to eight glasses of water per day; it flushes toxins from your body. Your digestive system needs water to function properly. Waste is flushed out in the form of urine and sweat. If you don't drink water, you don't flush out waste and it collects in your body, causing a myriad of problems. Water hydrates your body, which has a positive impact on your mood, your bodily performance and your skin.

Go for dark chocolate

Chocolates are loaded with sugar and caffeine. Dark chocolate, on the other hand, contains nutrients that can positively affect your health. Made from the seed of the cocoa tree, it is a great source of antioxidants. The catch is that you have to go for good quality dark chocolate with a high cocoa content.

Reap the benefits of lemons

Drinking water with lemon keeps your skin glowing, aids digestion, can help you lose weight, boosts your energy and is packed with vitamin C, which stimulates white blood cell production, vital for your immune system to function properly. Interestingly, lemon peels or rinds contain about five to ten times more vitamins than lemon juice. Grated lemon peel is a great addition to salads and teas. It adds amazing flavour.

Too much lemon can be bad for you. The acids in lemon juice can cause gastro-intestinal side-effects. Acidic foods may worsen symptoms of gastro-intestinal reflux disease, or GERD, and some people get an upset stomach when they consume too much ascorbic acid. Don't overdo it.

Go for probiotics

Probiotics are live bacteria and yeasts that are good for your digestive system. We usually think of bacteria as things that cause diseases, but your body is full of bacteria, both good and bad. Probiotics are often called "good" bacteria, because they help keep your gut healthy.

A very important lesson I learnt during my journey is that a healthy gut hosts a healthy immune system.

Our gut flora is the game changer in managing our immunity. To maintain a healthy immune system, you need to consider all the keys highlighted in this book. But should you not look after your gut, it will all be for nothing. One way to strengthen the gut is though probiotics. Plain Greek or Bulgarian yogurt with live cultures are great alternatives.

Limit your coffee intake

Coffee contains some essential nutrients and is high in antioxidants. Caffeine is a known stimulant. It thus increases your level of alertness. But as much as it can have a positive effect, these effects can be negative when you drink coffee at night. It might negatively impact your sleep patterns.

Having read many articles on this topic, I found that researchers have different opinions. My personal experience is that if I drink too much coffee it affects my digestion. If I limit my intake to two cups a day, I do not feel any negative side-effects.

It is worthwhile to mention that I have always battled with acid reflux and coffee does not help. I made one small change in my diet. My first cup of the day is rooibos tea instead of coffee. After that I allow myself one or two cups during the day. Amazingly, my acid reflux disappeared altogether.

It is important to remember that all these recommendations are general guidelines. They do not take into account any specific medical condition that you may have. Always consult your medical practitioner on what you should and should not eat if you have a specific condition.

Limit alcohol intake

According to the National Institute of Alcohol Abuse and Alcoholism (https://www.niaaa.nih.gov/alcohol-health/alcohols-effects-body), using alcohol can impact your brain, heart, liver, pancreas, immune system and sexual functioning.

The facts provided by the Health Promotion Agency in this article http://www.alcohol.org.nz/sites/default/files/documents/Body%20and%20health%20effects_MAY2015_web.pdf might shock you. If you suspect that you have a drinking problem, or would just like to know more, I highly recommend that you read this article.

Just note that while you are young, your body may be able to cope with the punishment you put it through, but as you age, the cumulative effects of bad habits will start catching up with you. Sadly, you may only realise what you have done to yourself when it is too late. Do not make this mistake! Read this article, and make a decision today to limit your alcohol intake.

Exercise

Aside from eating healthy food, another proactive step toward detoxing your body is regular exercise.

Exercise is probably the most important lever at your disposal to ensure that you proactively manage your stress.

In the South African context, most people think our only option is going to the gym. Running or cycling on the roads is not the safest choice. Unfortunately, most people I know do not like a gym. I have seen so many friends of mine (myself included) who wasted money on gym subscriptions after only going to the gym once or twice. Then we decided it was too much of a hassle. It takes too long to get there and even longer to get home. Let's just write it off as a bad debt.

Today I want to challenge you to think outside the box: Find out what works for you. Don't get hung up on traditional definitions of exercise. Climb the stairs at the office, take your dog for a walk in your townhouse complex or get a static cycling machine and cycle while you watch television.

When you experience stress, your body releases hormones such as cortisol, which have a negative impact on your immune system. Exercise helps reduce cortisol levels and increase feel good hormones such as serotonin, endorphins, adrenalin and dopamine.

Exercise, without your being aware of it, plays a significant role in detoxifying your body. For one, we sweat when we exercise. The body releases toxins through sweat. Secondly, as our heart rate increases, we breathe more heavily. Breathing is another great way of releasing toxins. The correct way to breathe is to breathe in through your nose and out through your mouth. I take my dogs for a daily walk. I try and concentrate on my breathing to rid my body from as much carbon dioxide as possible. Another habit I have acquired over the years is to do breathing exercises when I wake up and before I go to sleep. I breathe in through my nose for six seconds until my lungs are full, and then exhale slowly for about eight seconds. I repeat this about ten times. This is such a small activity you can engage in, but it will have a positive impact on your health.

If you have to choose one thing to do differently going into the future, I would say exercise. Besides the physical health benefits, it also has a dramatic impact on your emotional health. It is the best way of feeling better quickly. It also has a long-term effect on your overall health if you exercise regularly.

Sleep

One of the biggest threats of our day and age is lack of sleep. Prolonged stress and associated lack of sleep should be avoided at all cost. It is recommended that you should catch up on lost sleep within at least a week to prevent long-term damage to your body.

If you suffer from lack of sleep, the first step is to try and identify the cause. A typical cause, but one that is many times overlooked, is drinking stimulants in the evening. I am sure we all enjoy our favourite fizzy or alcoholic drink, coffee or chocolate in the evening. The caffeine can to keep you awake. If you want to drink something in the evening, stick to rooibos or herbal tea or caffeine-free cold drinks.

Late meals are another reason for failing to fall asleep. An attempt should always be made to eat by no later than 19h00. I facilitated workshops with a group of young professionals who were targeted as leaders of the future. A gentleman approached me on the issue of battling to fall asleep. After a few questions, I gathered that he eats supper at 22h00 in the evening and goes to bed straight after that.

After changing his supper time from 22h00 to 19h00, the problem was solved. What a relieved man.

A possible reason is exercise in the evening. Some people adjust well and can go to sleep after exercise. But this is not true for everyone. If you battle to fall asleep and you exercise in the evening, try exercising in the morning and see what happens.

A very common reason for lack of sleep is working too late. Most career driven people tend to take their work home. Given the nightmare traffic has become, many companies allow flexi-time. People start earlier and go home earlier. The negative effect is that most people still take their laptops home and work through their e-mails in the evening. If you work late, your brain is still very active. Therefore, once you go to bed, you are still trying to solve work problems and can't fall asleep.

Another common reason for lack of sleep is emotional distress. Most people, when going through any form of trauma, have difficulty falling asleep for a period after being exposed to the trauma. In a short space of time, I was mugged and we had a house break-in. I was literally too afraid to go to sleep. Every little sound woke me up. In severe cases, you may need to see your doctor who can prescribe sleeping tablets under his/her supervision. Taking tablets over the long-term is not a viable solution. Dealing with the fear is something you have to do. Go and see a psychologist who can help you work through your emotions.

If you suffer from sleeplessness and none of the above is affecting your sleep, you will need to look at addressing the root of your stress, whatever that may be in your case. Try and get to the bottom of it through elimination.

Many people that battle to sleep believe that reading a book or a magazine when going bed does the trick. Try it, it works for most people.

The bottom line is that you need rest for your body to recover. Without it your body will go into distress. **A good night's rest may literally clear the mind.**

Furthermore, your body cleanses itself while you sleep. The liver does a lot of its dirty work in the early morning hours. Pulling an all-nighter, or even staying up to watch a late-night show, will compromise the deeper sleep cycles that occur before midnight. Be sure to get up early as well, because you don't want to sleep through the hours when your body naturally wants to purge itself of waste. Letting your bowel movement fester, or holding back your urine until later in the morning can lead to it being reabsorbed by the body.

The moral of the story is that by getting a good night's sleep, you allow your body to detox naturally.

Relaxation and Self-expression

We know that relaxation is a necessity, not a luxury. We all need to relax to allow our bodies some recovery time. From a physiological point of view your body needs time out. So does your mind. Your body and mind detox when you take time out.

You might wonder why I combine relaxation and self-expression in one topic. The reality is that few people relax by purely throwing themselves onto a couch and doing nothing. The best way to relax is doing something in which you express yourself. For some people it means listening to music, watching television, others sing, or you may engage in some form of art or gardening. These are merely some examples. It all boils down to finding out what works for you. Women may not like this, but many men relax by playing computer games, golf or working on their toys (bikes, cars, four wheelers). Women often tend to prefer some form of art. You have to find out what works for you and do it. Having a goal is not enough; you need to put action to your words.

I need to qualify that relaxation is not the same as avoidance. Some people throw themselves into a specific activity to avoid what they need to face in their lives. That is not relaxation. Relaxation is an activity that will help you calm down at the end of the day and give you the strength and stamina to deal with your stress in a sustainable way.

Do this quick exercise. What hobbies do you currently have? What recreational activities do you participate in? My guess is that you are thinking about a couple of examples of things you used to do in the good old days. Before you go there, first think about what you do now. When you are done, think back what hobbies you used to enjoy? What recreational activities did you participate in which you do not have time for at the moment? What would you like to do in your spare time if you had any?

I am very fond of gardening. Whenever I have spent time in the garden getting my hands dirty, I feel like a different person. I have the pleasure of being outside in nature, it's a form of exercise and I clear my head. My other favourite pass time is cooking or baking. Every month after receiving my favourite magazine, I can't wait to try out a new recipe. What a pleasure! Make time for those activities that leave you feel relaxed. It won't happen by itself. You need to make it happen.

Recovery time

Recovery time is an interesting concept. It is closely related to relaxation. For the body to keep up with its challenges, it needs continual breaks that will allow it some recovery time. If you are studying, take a ten-minute break every two hours. You will note the difference in your ability to maintain the pace. If you work in an office, do the same. Take a walk outside and get some sun therapy (free Vitamin D injection). Just taking a few minutes' time out makes all the difference.

I know quite a few smokers who are quite healthy. This has puzzled me for a long time until I realised that every time they take a smoke break, they are getting recovery time. Make no mistake, I am not promoting smoking, I dislike it with a passion. The point is that taking regular short breaks could have a tremendous impact on your health and ability to cope with the daily stressors of life. Take time to smell the roses.

In summary on detoxing the body

Why wait for your body to be filled with toxins before you detox. This book does not focus on how to detox after the fact; the focus is rather on how to keep your body clean. Make a few simple lifestyle changes to achieve that. If you refrain from pumping your body full of toxins, your immune system will remain strong and able to deal with most things that are thrown at it. The best way to manage stress is to do so proactively!

Chapter 8 - Build your house on a Rock

"The purpose of life is to live a life of purpose." Richard Leider

The fourth key is building your house on a Rock. As was mentioned in Chapter 3, building your house on a rock essentially means that you have a spiritual belief which provides you with solid ground to stand on. If you do not build your house on the Rock, your life will be aimless and without purpose. The knowledge that there is a higher power which is in control and looks out for you, gives you the strength to deal with life's ups and downs.

In my case Jesus is my Rock. In Jeremiah 29:10 of the New International Version of the Bible, the Lord says: "For I know the plans I have for you, plans to prosper you and not to harm you, plans to give you hope and a future."

Find your purpose

People who have a clear purpose in their lives tend to be happier and experience less stress. They know the hardship they experience will eventually have a good result. As was said in the introduction, if you are a boat floating aimlessly at sea, you will be stressed. You will feel as though your life is meaningless. You will feel uncertain. You will fear the future. On the other hand, if you steer that boat in a direction of your choice, you will feel in control. You will experience a sense of purpose. All the anxiety of not knowing where you are going will evaporate!

Make an effort to find your purpose and set goals. Even if you don't achieve them as you planned, it still gives you a target to work towards. Life is funny; it often throws a curveball or two. You may be steering your boat to beautiful island. On the way you will inevitably be thrown off course by a storm or two. You may even decide to change direction. The island you were planning to go to may have had too many sharks in the water. As a result, you can decide to head for another island. That is okay.

The only reason we have a plan is to be able to deviate from it. That's life. But having a plan gives us purpose and direction. Make those plans, but be flexible enough to deviate from them and head in a different direction if required.

How do we find our purpose? Let me take you through a process that will help you get there.

Values

Let's start with your values. Consider the list below and indicate which of these values you aspire to and which do you reject.

Values	Aspire to	Reject
Excellence		
Tolerance		
Adrenalin rush		
Looking out for myself		
Integrity		
Making a difference		
Live life today!		
Pleasing others		
Pursuit of happiness		
Being there for others when they need me		
Winning!		
Continuous improvement		
Spiritual growth		
Be respected professionally		

Values	Aspire to	Reject
Be a good partner/spouse/parent		
Be an effective leader		
Personal growth		
Accomplishing personal goals		
Emotional security		
Give myself freely in helping others		
Material wealth		
Getting along with others		
Security		
Dependable		
Authenticity		
Optimism/enthusiasm		
Balance		
Other – if you have another, please add!		

Now take some time to consider whom you admire and why? Also consider whom you dislike and why?

Keep a piece of paper handy and make some notes.

Once you have done this, consider what you spend your time on?

Here is a list of typical activities:

Examples of Activities
Work
Personal development
Relationships/socialisation (romance, family, friends)
Exercise
Recreation/fun
Sleep
Intellectual development
Spiritual development
"Me" time (I am at the centre of my universe)
Finances
Healthy eating
Unhealthy eating
Travel
Other?

Assign percentages to each of these activities, ensuring that the various elements add up to 100. Once you have completed this exercise, consider what you want your spouse, your parents, children (if you have any), friends and colleagues to say at your funeral. Tackle them each individually. This exercise will take you to the heart of who you would like to be.

Considering what you mentioned above in terms of your values, what you admire in others and what you want said at your funeral, how does that match with what you spend your time on? Too often when I do this exercise with people, they admit that their values are, for instance, to be a good friend or partner, being there for others, but in reality, they focus on acquiring "stuff" and working day and night. So, what happens in practice? The values they aspire to is not what they are living day by day. Where are you? What are your values and where is your disconnect, if any?

My guess is that there may be a gap between what you value and what you spend your time on. Don't be alarmed. It is quite common. Few people take the time to think about what they value and challenge themselves whether they actually live up to it. This book is all about creating an awareness of where you are in your life and where you would like to be. By creating the awareness that you may be valuing one thing and doing another, the battle is half won. All you need to do now is take accountability and do something about it.

Brand

Now let's take it a step further. Let's consider your brand. Yes, organisations do have brands, but without realising it, each one of us also has a brand by which people know and recognise us. A brand helps you differentiate yourself from others, it creates visibility and loyalty for the unique package you offer your customers and clients. It helps you attract people and opportunities. And ultimately it helps you achieve your goals. Complete the following sentences about yourself:

I am...
I believe in...
I treasure...
My actions speak of...
I enjoy spending time on...
I would like to...

For a moment put yourself in the shoes of your family, friends or co-workers. What do they recognise you for? What do they see as your brand?

Given your answers to the above, what do you think is your brand? You should always try and limit the description of your brand to one or at the most three words. My own brand for instance is "Just done it". Everyone who knows me knows that I like getting things done. So what is yours?

Now that you understand your values and your brand, let's consider passion.

Passion

Mihaly Csikszentmihalyi (1995) is the originator of the concept of "FLOW". He said that we must have a conviction that our lives serve a useful purpose and has value. Money, security and comfort are important, but not enough. Have you ever felt exhilarated when doing something?

He says FLOW is the feeling of exhilaration that you experience when you do something that you have a passion for. At such a time you are completely focused and determined, moving effortlessly with high energy, drawn into the complexity of the task, passionately involved and all that matter is the present.

Now take a moment to consider when you felt like this? TD Jakes (https://za.pinterest.com/pin/540643130238456539/) said, "If you can't figure out your purpose, figure out your passion. For your passion will lead you right to your purpose."

By taking time to meditate on your values, brand and passion, you should get much closer to knowing what your purpose is. My purpose in life is to make a difference in people's lives. If I get too busy worrying about myself or things in my life that may detract my attention, I consciously pull myself back and ask myself what would God want me to do? Whose life does he want me to touch? The moment I focus on helping others, my life gets meaning and I tend to fret less about my own issues.

Let go and let God

Jesus said, "Come to me, all you who are weary and burdened, and I will give you rest. Take my yoke upon you and learn from me, for I am gentle and humble in heart, and you will find rest for your souls. For my yoke is easy and my burden is light" (Matthew 11:28–30). The ultimate solution for those currently experiencing burnout is to find refreshment in Christ. For those with a particularly high level of burnout, this refreshment may include obtaining medical support and drastically altering their lifestyles. Others may find refreshment through seeing a counsellor. Reading encouraging scriptures (such as Romans 8, John 15 or Psalm 139) can be life altering.

Faith starts with hope. In Chapter 2 we spoke about detoxing your mind and keeping your thoughts focused on the positives in your life. If you have a negative outlook on life, nothing good will ever happen. But if you believe that good things are coming your way, you will draw it like a magnet.

Romans 15:13 reads "May the God of hope fill you with all joy and peace as you trust in Him, so that you may overflow with hope by the power of the Holy Spirit."

Keep your eye on God and trust that He is in control. He has a great plan for your life. The question is how do we get there? It is by being faithful and doing your bit while God is setting things in motion. Be good and do good.

Mathew 6:33 reads: "But seek first His kingdom and His righteousness, and all these things will be given to you as well." We tend to focus so much on ourselves and what we want, have and don't have. Stop right there, first seek the kingdom of God and His righteousness.

This means that you need to build a relationship with God. Spend time with God and spend time in the Word. He will guide your every step.

And when things get tough, look up and thank the Lord for all He has done for you, for all the blessings in your life. Thank Him for all the blessings that are to come and for His favours in your life.

Wake up thanking Him and go to bed thanking Him.

Let's consider the story of Joseph, courtesy Wikipedia.
Joseph was the son of Jacob (Israel) and Rachel, who lived in Canaan with eleven brothers and one sister. He was Rachel's firstborn and Jacob's eleventh son and his father's favourite. His half-brothers hated him for this.

When Joseph was seventeen, he had two dreams that led to his demise. In the first dream Joseph and his brothers gathered bundles of grain. Then all of the grain bundles that had been prepared by the brothers gathered around Joseph's bundle and bowed down to it. In the second dream, the sun (father), the moon (mother) and eleven stars (brothers) bowed down to Joseph himself. When he told these dreams to his brothers, they were angered by the implication that the family would bow down to him (Genesis 37:1-11). They then plotted to kill him, but instead, sold him to traders on their way to Egypt and told their father that Joseph was killed by wild animals.

In Egypt Joseph was sold to Potiphar, the captain of Pharaoh's guard. While serving in Potiphar's household, God was with Joseph, so he prospered and became superintendent. Potiphar's wife desired

Joseph and tried to seduce him, but he resisted. Angered, she falsely claimed the reverse and Joseph was imprisoned (Genesis 39:1-20).

In prison Joseph interpreted the dreams of two of Pharaoh's senior servants. Two years later Pharaoh had two dreams which disturbed him, and when none of his wise men could interpret them, Joseph was summoned.

He explained that Pharaoh's dreams foretold seven years of abundance, followed by seven years of famine and he advised Pharaoh to store surplus grain during the years of abundance. When the famine came, it was so severe that people from surrounding nations ("from all over the earth") came to Egypt to buy bread, as this nation was the only one prepared for the seven-year drought.

During the famine, Joseph's brothers went to Egypt to buy grain. There they bowed before Joseph, the Vizier, but did not recognise him. However, Joseph recognised them, but disguised himself. He accused them of being spies. After they mentioned that they had left a younger brother, Benjamin, at home, Joseph demanded that Benjamin be brought to Egypt as a demonstration of their veracity. So they left for Canaan.

After they had consumed all the grain they brought from Egypt, the brothers had to go back to Egypt for more, this time accompanied by Benjamin. Upon their return to Egypt, Joseph revealed himself as their brother. He had their father brought to Egypt, so they were all reunited.

Every time I feel disheartened, I think of Joseph. He never lost sight of seeking the Kingdom of God and he reaped every single benefit, eventually. Through all his trials and tribulations, God was working His plan in Joseph's favour. Joseph never strayed, but kept his eye on God.

This is a decision you need to make for yourself, I just know that without God in my life, directing my every move, my life would be devoid of meaning. I would not be able to cope with the trials of life. But what I do know is, with God on my side, I can conquer anything and everything!

What are your spiritual beliefs? Do you have a higher power which you can count on, where you can be safe, and who will help you carry your burdens?

Chapter 9 - Ensuring lasting change

There are two primary choices in life: to accept conditions as they are, or accept the responsibility for changing them.

What now?

By now you have significantly raised your self-awareness. You should know what your stressors are and be clear on what negative thoughts you need to replace with positive ones. You should have a good idea of what environmental toxins are compromising your health. And you should have clarity on food and drink choices impacting your health.

Most importantly, you will know whether your house is built on a Rock or on sand. In this case, a decision and action is required on your part.

By now you know what you must do. The question is how do you make these changes and ensure that they last?

In this chapter, you will be provided with some practical steps you can take to make the change in your life last a lifetime. I will also share with you some of my own experiences and the changes I made in my life towards sustainable health.

Know your priorities

We all complain about not having enough time. Regardless what we do, no day will have more than 24 hours. You can't do it all. You need to decide on your priorities. To have a good understanding of your priorities, you need to know what you value in life.

It is very important that you realise that your priorities differ, depending where you are in your life. This is where the concept work-life-balance comes in. If you are a young professional climbing the corporate ladder, you are likely to spend more of your time on your career. You may consciously decide to put romantic relationships and family on the back burner. What you can never afford to put on the back burner is your health. No matter what priorities you have at any given time in your life, you need to look after yourself. By keeping healthy, you will be able to handle anything.

In the introduction, I mentioned that there is a tendency today to try and keep all the balls in the air. That is not feasible. You are only one person.

You need to manage your time. And managing your time is based on your current priorities.

If you have recently suffered from an illness which severely affected you, your priority would be to build you immune system and get healthy. That may mean that your career moves to second place.

I could quote multiple examples, but I think by now you have the message. You need to keep in touch with yourself and your changing priorities and make sure that the things you spend your time on reflect your priorities. If not, it may add to your stress levels. You will feel guilty for not doing everything you should be doing, which will have a severe impact on your stress levels.

As your priorities change, allow yourself to focus on what is important to you at that point in time.

You can repeat this exercise every few months to quickly check whether you are still on track and to help you continuously and consciously prioritise.

Habits

We all have our weaknesses. Mine is comfort food. Some people escape using alcohol, others smoke, and some use drugs. Reality is that all of these could cumulatively kill you over time.

Let's take alcohol abuse. Alcohol depletes vitamin B from your body and changes your body's metabolism, for some people more than others. Using alcohol can be addictive. Through continuous use, it eventually destroys brain and liver cells which cause difficulty in concentration.

Smoking (nicotine) affects the oxygen flow in your blood and thus negatively affects body cells. It depletes vitamin C from your body. It also dulls the brain. And ladies, in case you did not know, it does cause wrinkles. Smoking is a major cause of heart disease, cancer, emphysema and colds.

Given our incredibly rushed lifestyles, we need to cope at all times. As a result, we tend to turn to painkillers more often than is good for us. The overuse of Paracetamol-based painkillers is toxic to the liver. Painkillers can cause digestive problems.

I don't like using this example, because it is one of my weaknesses, but too much coffee is not good for you. One or two cups a day is fine. You need to know that especially when you are stressed, you need to avoid adrenalin stimulants such as coffee and chocolate (I'm guilty of both). They wreak havoc with your blood glucose levels, aggravate heartburn and will make your irritable bowel worse. Caffeine is also a diuretic. That is why you are often warned that drinking too much coffee leads to dehydration.

All these bad habits put strain on your body, which impacts your ability to deal with stress. A healthy body is much more able to sustain constant stress and pressure, than one that is loaded with toxins.

Whatever you use to escape, just know that habits can become addictions, and addictions will harm you. You know your poor habits. Get yourself informed.

Know what you are doing to yourself and do something about it!

But remember that to change a habit you need to consistently replace your bad habit with a good one for at least 21 consecutive days, after which the new habit will take root. We will talk more about habits in the next chapter.

First you need to understand the dynamics of habits. There are good habits and bad ones. Regardless what anyone may tell you, it is much easier to develop a bad habit than it is to develop a good habit. One can learn a bad habit over night, but it takes at least three weeks (21 consecutive days) to develop a good habit. If you want to have fool proof success, keep it up for six weeks. For instance, if you started a new habit such as a daily walk and you skip one day, you need to start again at day one. Otherwise you will run the risk of falling back into your old habits. Good habits are only set in concrete if you practice them religiously for three to six weeks every day. You only need to do this for the first month or so, after that, even if you deviate from your habit, you will feel the instinctive need to go back to it. Because people differ, some establish habits quicker than others. To be on the safe side, keep it up for six weeks.

Many years ago I vowed to live a healthier life. One of the habits I had to master was drinking six to eight glasses of water every day. At that stage I was lucky if I drank one glass a day. To make it easier on myself, and having studied the dynamics of habits, I started drinking a glass of water with every other drink I had. Every time I drank a cup of coffee, I also drank a glass of water. For every glass of wine I had, I drank a glass of water. I also decided to drink a glass of water with every meal I ate. By linking the water to existing habits that had already been established, I made it much easier for myself. After three meals and three cups of coffee, I already reached my minimum quota of water for the day. I am happy to say that to this day I am addicted to water. As I am sitting here in front of my laptop, I have my bottle of water next to the computer.

Please realise that you can't lose or drop a habit. Your best chance of getting rid of a bad habit is replacing it with another habit. For example, if you want to stop smoking, you'll need to exchange your smoking habit with another habit, such as sucking on a mint. Or my favourite subject: if you want to quit eating too many chocolates, you need to replace it with something healthy such as nuts or fruit. If you try to just quit without replacing the bad habit with a good one, the chances are 99% you will go back to your bad habit. The process, as with everything else, starts with self-awareness. You need to know what you want or need to change. You may not always be keen to let go of your bad habits, but sometimes you do not have a choice, especially when your health suffers as result of your poor habits. To get back to my water drinking example: I soon replaced drinking coffee almost altogether with drinking water instead.

The last bit of advice I would like to give you on habits is to choose your words. For example, instead of telling yourself and everyone else that you want to "give up" smoking, rather say that you would like to "free yourself from this bad habit for your own good". It will also help align your thinking, which will help you persevere in your quest.

Remember to link new habits to existing behaviour patterns or habits. Routine is very important. Routine removes stress and brings a sense of being in control. Replace bad habits with good ones. And choose your words in changing your habits.

By now I am sure you have a very good idea as to your bad habits. You may have denied some of it in the past, but you are slowly realising that denial won't do you any good. If you have identified more than one habit you would like to change or nurture, then the next section is just for you.

Linking habits back to our four keys, you can now define which habits you wish to develop aligned with each of the keys. Do you need to replace negative thoughts with constructive ones? What environmental toxins can you remove from your life? How can you change your eating and drinking habits to support your body? What habits do you need to cultivate to develop your spiritual life? Only you can define these.

Be realistic, yet specific

The single biggest mistake we make is trying to change too much at once. Prioritise what you want to achieve through lifestyle changes. Define what habits can help you and then start with the most important one.

Tackle one major change at a time.

Too much change is overwhelming. You could set yourself up for failure. But do not lose sight of all four keys. Be sure to make changes in all four areas of your life.

If you need to stop smoking, drink less coffee, start eating better, and start exercising, it will be too much to tackle at once. If your life fits this scenario and you are overweight as well, I would start with changing my eating habits. You will lose weight much quicker by eating well than starting to exercise. Once you have your eating habits mastered, you can move on to exercise. Once you start exercising, you may want to stop smoking just because you want to.

The second biggest mistake people make is setting unachievable goals.

Take baby steps. Set realistic targets which you will achieve.

If you were used to take-away food every night, don't think you can start off by replacing all your junk food with healthy wholesome meals. Take baby steps. Start of by replacing every second day's meal with a healthy home-made meal. You can even, when ordering take-out, consider choosing a healthier option on the menu, like grilled chicken instead of deep fried chicken.

Set yourself achievable targets!

How will you know whether you can achieve your goals? *You need to set clear, measurable targets.* If you currently eat junk food five times a week, have a clear goal of reducing that to three times a week in the first week, and twice a week in the second week, and once a week after that. Set yourself a target to eat at least three meals a day and not skip a meal. For the first two weeks, at least one meal per day should be healthy, i.e. low fat protein and vegetables or salad. These are clear, measurable goals. Now set you own targets. Be as specific as you can.

Buddy up

By now you have prioritised the lifestyle changes you want to make to achieve long-term health and optimal performance. You have defined realistic goals and know what habits you want to cultivate. Now you need to buddy up.

When we set out on a path to develop new habits, the road is bumpy, full of diversions and often very steep.

By finding yourself a buddy to support you in your quest, you build in a safety mechanism that will protect you against giving up.

The best example is exercise, especially when you are in the first three to six-week period of acquiring a new habit. That is when you desperately need a buddy. A few years back I travelled a lot for work. I started using it as an excuse not to exercise. Soon I was not in the mood for any physical exercise. I have always believed in regular exercise. My travelling tapered down and I decided to re-establish by exercise habit. The first month I went to the gym. By paying for it, I felt compelled to go. My intent was that the first month would be my four weeks in which I would establish my habit, after which I would keep it up at home.

After two weeks of religious exercise, my travelling started again. I knew how critical it was not to stop. I worked out a home routine which I did every evening that I spent away from home. After two weeks in the gym, I realised I really enjoyed the mini trampoline, as well as the ball exercises. I already had a treadmill at home, as well as a stepper and a few exercise DVDs. When I was at home, I alternated my exercise routines. Some people can do the same type of exercise every day. It has two downsides. One, your body gets used to the type of exercise and you see results at a much slower rate. Secondly, you get bored. I get bored very easily. I therefore need to ensure I do not do the same exercise routine more than twice a week. I try and exercise at least five times per week. Once you have established your routine, you will soon see that you cannot live without it. After I left the gym, I continued to exercise after work with a friend of mine. She only lasted three weeks, but between my two weeks at the gym, and three weeks with my friend, it gave me enough time to properly root my new habit.

If you have decided to establish exercise as a habit, or in other words as a lifestyle change, just make sure you nurture this habit long enough to make sure that it sticks. Start today! You will never be sorry. And if you are tackling exercise or dieting in particular, find a buddy. Get someone who will stand by your side and provide the peer pressure you need.

Enjoy

I've said this before, but it bears repeating. You must enjoy the lifestyle changes your make to help you proactively combat stress. Do exercises you enjoy. Find fun ways of expressing yourself. Make your daily environment a fun place to be in. Listen to your favourite music. Expose yourself to relationships you enjoy. Set healthy boundaries. Enjoy your journey.

Non-negotiables

Let me summarise the recipe for successful proactive stress management. If you follow my advice, you will sustain a high level of performance and good health even when the stressors you are exposed to are excessive.

Considering the four keys of avoiding burnout and achieving sustainable health, the following are most critical:
1. Detox the mind – take hold of your thoughts and get rid of all the toxic ones.
2. Detox the environment – remove as many toxins from your immediate environment as you can. Replace them with non-toxic alternatives.
3. Detox the body – eat well, drink enough water, sleep well and exercise regularly.
4. Build your house on a Rock – find your spiritual foundation.

It is as simple as that. If you don't compromise any one of these, you will bear the fruit!

My guess is that at the end of this chapter you may feel a bit overwhelmed with everything you've learned. Your self-awareness has been raised significantly. You've identified a host of actions you need to take to manage your stress proactively. Do not despair, prioritise and start with the important lifestyle changes.

My story

Detox the mind

I have always known the importance of channelling my thoughts and avoiding toxic thoughts. But after I was diagnosed with Graves Disease, I was sick for a long time. During this time, I first had hyperthyroidism, which raised my heart rate significantly. This left me exhausted, so much so that I battled to get out of bed. I could do nothing. Then, after receiving the radioactive iodine treatment, my whole body went into a toxic state for months. My eyes were swollen, my legs and body were swollen, and I gained 10kg. I looked and felt terrible, but no doctor could help me. My GP told me that it was in my head and that the blood tests showed no abnormalities. Then I started reading up on natural ways to strengthen my immune system. I also managed to find an endocrinologist who was willing to assist me all the way. He did the right blood tests and found that many of my hormones were either elevated or too low. I started using the correct medicine and natural supplements and changed my whole lifestyle. Within three weeks I was a different person. It took me a few months to get into remission, but by now I could move in the right direction. During this time, my thought patterns went for a loop. I constantly thought I would never get better. I thought that this was a life sentence.

I realised one day that I needed to check my thoughts. I started to consciously and actively control my thoughts. When I woke up in the morning, I would declare that I am healthy and would thank the Lord for guiding me to complete health. I have this habit to this day.

I also make great effort to allow no negative and toxic thoughts to mull in my mind. Whenever toxic thoughts try to take hold of me, I remind myself that everything works out for the best. God is in control and I have nothing and no one to fear. He has my best interest at heart.

I need to add that changing your thoughts is one of the hardest things to do. But you know what, it is possible. And once you are in the habit of killing toxic thoughts before they can take root, it becomes easier. Eventually it becomes like driving your car. You need not think about it, it just happens. It's worth noting that changing thoughts are also changing habits. In other words, you need to do so consistently for few weeks.

Detox the environment

After I started reading up on toxins in my environment, I soon realised that this would be an area where I had lots of work to do. Luckily these changes are easier to make.

I started off by getting rid of all pesticides. I grow my own vegetables and it was crucial to stay away from toxic fumes and poisons in my garden. I use natural alternatives for all fungi and pests. The internet has various recipes for natural alternatives. My favourite for fungus growth on my vegetables is chamomile tea. I just spray once or twice a week. Chilli pepper and garlic sprays are also quite popular. As an insecticide for indoors, I use an Efekto product called Bio Kill Classic. It is odourless and biodegradable. I also use it for ants inside and outside the house. This product is amazing!

Next I replaced all my air fresheners in the house with natural alternatives. I never realised just how toxic air fresheners were until I replaced them with natural alternatives.

In Chapter 6 we explored all the toxic household chemicals. I chose to replace all household cleaning chemicals with Pick n Pay's green range. I use the kitchen and bathroom cleaners, window cleaner, degreaser, toilet cleaner and dish washing liquid. I use their degreaser as a tile cleaner. Dischem's Eco Home dishwashing liquid works really well.

After I eliminated all the above, I realised that washing detergent affected me. I wish I realised this earlier! I replaced washing powder with Bicarbonate of Soda. It is so effective I do not need to use a fabric softener.

Another product that wreaked havoc with my body was furniture polish. I replaced it with coconut oil. Using only a little bit has an incredibly nourishing effect on wood.

By now you can see that this was quite a process. It did not happen overnight. It probably took me eight to ten months to make all these changes. Next I replaced all my facial cleaning products with natural alternatives made of rooibos. Then all my make-up was replaced with the BioNikeDefence range.

One product I almost oversaw was sunscreen. Trust me, sunscreen is extremely toxic. Get a non-toxic alternative from your health shop or local pharmacy. And obviously, I replaced my favourite perfume with a natural alternative that I make myself, using essential oils.

Needless to say, as we get older we need to keep those grey hairs at bay! I replaced my hair colour with a version without ammonia and other harsh chemicals. Dischem has a great range.

Let's not forget about toothpaste. Fluoride interferes with thyroid function. I make my own toothpaste by combining coconut oil and bicarbonate of soda into a paste. Non-toxic alternatives are also available from health shops.

Lastly, I replaced all my water bottles and plastic containers with glass ones. I still have some plastic containers, but they are BPA free. My pots and pans are now cast iron, stainless steel or ceramic. Out with the non-stick!

Detox the body

I stopped drinking tap water. I use water from a reputable supplier that is free of chloride.

Especially if you have an autoimmune disease, it is worth removing sugar and gluten from your diet. These two changes had a significant impact on improving my health. Every now and again I let myself go and have some crisps and chocolates. But trust me, my body very quickly tells me to stop.

I only use Himalayan salt and fresh herbs from my garden. To avoid buying vegetables contaminated with pesticides, I started my own vegetable garden. I regularly make and eat bone broth. It is loaded with minerals that support the immune system and heals the gut lining and reduces intestinal inflammation.

Another significant toxin is alcohol. As much as I enjoy a glass of wine, I need to keep it to the bare minimum. I limit my dairy intake.

I drink six to eight glasses of water a day and start my day with rooibos tea. I try and limit my coffee intake. This helps a lot with my acid levels.

I try and eat at least two portions of vegetables each day, one fruit and give preference to white meat. I limit my carbohydrate intake, but when I do eat them, I stick to complex carbohydrates.

One healthy habit I started was drinking a plain yogurt smoothie in the morning with berries and ground flaxseed. The probiotics in the yogurt, combined with the potent antioxidants of dark berries and the anti-inflammatory properties of flaxseed, is a great way to start the day. Another great snack during the day is dried goji berries, again loaded with antioxidants.

I exercise daily. During summer, I swim in the morning and evening and right through the year I take my dogs for a long walk in the afternoon. As mentioned before, exercise is a great way to rid the body of toxins. My dogs are my buddies. It is so funny; they beg to go for a walk. Sometimes I run late. They then come and wag their tails and prompt me to go. I have noticed that when I feel tired and lethargic, that is the best time to go for a walk or a run. I feel like a different person afterwards.

I go out of my way to make sure my bedroom setup is such that I get a good night's sleep. No noise, fresh air, limited light. I also try to eat dinner at 18h00 and avoid eating after 19h00.

Let me say one last word on detoxing the body. My endocrinologist introduced me to a fantastic natural product, namely dandelion herb/root cut. It is sold in the form a tea. This tea is regarded as one of the best herbs to treat kidney and liver illnesses. It reduces fluid retention and removes toxins from the body. It comes highly recommended!

Build your house on a Rock

I start my day by watching a church service on satellite television or reading my Bible. I also make an effort to talk to God before my day starts, thanking him for all the blessings in my life and my good health.

Furthermore, I try to make a difference in the lives of others. There are people that I have built a relationship with over many years and I try my best to be there for them, to make a difference where I can. Others cross my path and when I get that feeling that I need to lend a helping hand, I do.

In Closing

Every single change makes a difference! You just need to start somewhere.

Where are you today? What are your biggest stressors? How are you coping with it? What can you do to avoid burnout? How can you use the four keys?

Remember, the aim is to achieve sustainable performance through proactive stress management.

Raise your self-awareness, take accountability for your life, and take action! The ball is now in your court...

Romans 12:11-17 in the Message translation summarises it beautifully:
"11 Don't burn out; keep yourselves fuelled and aflame. Be alert servants of the Master,
12 Cheerfully expectant. Don't quit in hard times; pray all the harder.
13 Help needy Christians; be inventive in hospitality.
14 Bless your enemies; no cursing under your breath.
15 Laugh with your happy friends when they're happy; share tears when they're down.
16 Get along with each other; don't be stuck-up. Make friends with nobodies; don't be the great somebody.
17 Don't hit back; discover beauty in everyone."

References

American Heart Association. (2015). *Smoking: Do you really know the risks?* [Online] Available at: http://www.heart.org/HEARTORG/HealthyLiving/QuitSmoking/QuittingSmoking/Smoking-Do-you-really-know-the-risks_UCM_322718_Article.jsp#.WG93oXdh0dU. [Accessed 10 Dec. 2016].

American Heart Association. (2015). *Why should I limit sodium?* [Online] Available at: https://www.heart.org/idc/groups/heart-public/@wcm/@hcm/documents/downloadable/ucm_300625.pdf. [Accessed 10 Oct. 2016].

Bauer, B.A. (2016). *What is BPA, and what are the concerns about BPA?* [Online] Available at: http://www.mayoclinic.org/healthy-lifestyle/nutrition-and-healthy-eating/expert-answers/bpa/faq-20058331. [Accessed 7 Jan. 2017].

Campaign for Safe Cosmetics. (2017). *Chemicals of concern.* [Online] Available at: http://www.safecosmetics.org/get-the-facts/chemicals-of-concern/. [Accessed 10 Dec. 2016].

Campbell, T. (2014). *12 Frightening Facts about Milk.* [Online] Available at: http://nutritionstudies.org/12-frightening-facts-milk/. [Accessed 4 Jan. 2017].

Chapman, G. (2010). *The 5 love languages.* 4th Ed. United States of America: Northfield Publishing.

Cleveland Clinic. (2014). *That Cosy Fire Could Be Hazardous to Your Health.* [Online] Available at: https://health.clevelandclinic.org/2014/12/that-cozy-fire-could-be-hazardous-to-your-health/. [Accessed 1 Dec. 2016].

Cook, M.S. (2014). *10 Toxic ingredients lurking in common perfumes and colognes.* [Online] Available at: http://www.care2.com/greenliving/10-toxic-ingredients-lurking-in-common-perfumes-and-colognes.html. [Accessed 8 Jan. 2017].

Corriher, S.C. (2009). *How air fresheners are killing you.* [Online] Available at: http://healthwyze.org/reports/184-how-air-fresheners-are-killing-you. [Accessed 3 Jan. 2017].

Csikszentmihalyi, M. (2016). *The pursuit of happiness.* [Online] Available at: http://www.pursuit-of-happiness.org/history-of-happiness/mihaly-csikszentmihalyi/. [Accessed 10 Jan. 2017].

Dr Axe. (2016). *77 Coconut Oil Uses & Cure.* [Online] Available at: https://draxe.com/coconut-oil-uses/. [Accessed 10 Oct. 2016].

Dr Axe. (n.d.) *Top 10 natural sweeteners and sugar alternatives.* [Online] Available at: https://draxe.com/natural-sweeteners/. [Accessed 17 Dec. 2016].

Dr. Group, E. (2016). *12 Toxins in Your Drinking Water.* [Online] Available at: http://www.globalhealingcenter.com/natural-health/12-toxins-in-your-drinking-water/. [Accessed 6 Jan. 2017].

Dr. Hyman. (2010). *Dairy: 6 Reasons You Should Avoid it at all Costs.* [Online] Available at: http://drhyman.com/blog/2010/06/24/dairy-6-reasons-you-should-avoid-it-at-all-costs-2/. [Accessed 7 Jan. 2017].

Dr Leaf. (n.d.) *Controlling your toxic thoughts.* [Online] Available at: http://drleaf.com/about/toxic-thoughts/. [Accessed 3 Jan. 2017].

Environmental Working Group. (n.d.) [Online] Available at: http://www.ewg.org/research/healthy-home-tips/tip-6-skip-non-stick-avoid-dangers-teflon. [Accessed 15 Dec. 2016].

Jakes, T.D. (n.d.) [Online] https://za.pinterest.com/pin/540643130238456539/ [Accessed 5 Jan. 2017]

James, M. (2016). *Safe dish soap guide.* [Online] Available at: https://gimmethegoodstuff.org/safe-product-guides/dish-soap/. [Accessed 4 Jan. 2017].

Mamavation. (n.d.) *What's that smell? What toxins lurk in your favorite perfumes?* [Online] Available at: http://mamavation.com/2015/03/toxic-perfume-chemicals.html. [Accessed 12 Nov. 2016].

Markham, D. (2016). *8 Natural & homemade insecticides to save your garden without killing the earth.* [Online] Available at: http://www.treehugger.com/lawn-garden/8-natural-homemade-insecticides-save-your-garden-without-killing-earth.html. [Accessed 4 Jan. 2017].

Morehouse, D. (n.d.) *Cell phones and Remote Viewers.* [Online] Available at: http://www.bibliotecapleyades.net/scalar_tech/esp_scalartech27.htm. [Accessed 8 Jan. 2017].

National Institute of Alcohol abuse and alcoholism. (n.d.) *Alcohol's Effects on the Body.* [Online] Available at: https://www.niaaa.nih.gov/alcohol-health/alcohols-effects-body. [Accessed 7 Jan. 2017].

National Institutes of Health. (2013). *Brain may flush out toxins during sleep.* [Online] Available at: https://www.nih.gov/news-events/news-releases/brain-may-flush-out-toxins-during-sleep. [Accessed 15 Dec. 2016].

New International Version Holy Bible. (2011). 4th Ed. United States of America: Zondervan.

Organics. (n.d.) *Table Salt vs. Himalayan Pink Salt: What's the Difference?* [Online] Available at: http://organics.org/table-salt-vs-himalayan-sea-salt-whats-the-difference/. [Accessed 20 Dec. 2016].

Palkhivala, A. (2001). *Stressed Out? Don't Let It Become Burnout.* [Online] Available at: http://www.webmd.com/balance/stress-management/news/20010815/stressed-out-dont-let-become-burnout. [Accessed 12 Dec. 2016].

Rabkin, J.G. and Struening, E.L. (1976). Life Events, Stress and Illness. *Science*, (194), pp. 1013-1020.

Wikipedia. (2016). *Holmes & Rahe stress scale.* [Online] Available at: https://en.wikipedia.org/wiki/Holmes_and_Rahe_stress_scale. [Accessed 2 Dec. 2016].